Fat Loss The Truth
Why the medical research might just shock you

Dr. John Fitzgerald

D1473878

Fat Loss The Truth
ISBN-13: 978-1463780852
ISBN-10:1463780850
Copyright © 2012 by John Fitzgerald

For years, John F Kennedy wouldn't eat lunch and he would get so thin.

Jackie Kennedy

I like to laugh and joke around. Most of the time I am joking around. So if you find anything in this book that sounds offensive, realize it is coming from me and is meant to put a smile on your face. ☺ I will make fun of anything I can at anytime I can. It's just the way I am, If you can't make fun of others, who can you make fun of...right? ☺ Notice, if you see a smiley face, relax and laugh because it's good for you.

Einstein said that if you can't explain it to a 6 yr old, you don't understand it yourself. The greatest challenge I had writing this book was keeping it simple. Since I am not as smart as Einstein was, I had my 12-year-old take part in the editing of this book.

I wrote this book with many simple stories so that anyone can understand it, not just doctors. This is a great book for doctors to give to their patients, all their patients.

Magazines commonly have articles that say you need to eat every 3 or 4 or 5 hours to get lean. Or you may have heard that nibbling all day long is the key to losing weight...really...how about not eating all day?

Just use the common sense that you had before your head was filled with dieting and nutrition false knowledge. You may have to go back and ask someone whose head is not full of ridiculous food statements.

Just as a test, I asked my 7 year old..."Logan, do you see that big fat guy over there?"

"Yes"

"Well, do you think he got fat from not eating"

"No, he ate too much"

My point is, even a child knows this simple fact. Yet, fitness magazines will tell you something else. Maybe the fat guy ate too high a percentage of carbs or fat…or God forbid, maybe the fat guy didn't have a protein shake every 3 hours.

The more complicated an eating plan is, the less likely people will follow it.

The more complicated the explanations, the more people fade out and are less likely to read it and miss the whole big picture.

Contents

1   Opening Thought

"A good book should be more than the sum of its words. It should provoke thought and leave you with a gift that has the ability to change you forever."

Dr. John Fitzgerald

When I was young I had a firm grasp of the obvious. The obvious being that if I skipped some meals, I leaned up.

This remained obvious until I had been in practice for a while.

Then, fat loss suddenly became so much more complicated with the Body for Life bodybuilding diet eating 6 meals per day, the Zone Diet, eating low fat and high carb, eating raw, eating low carb, high fat, taking fat loss supplements, becoming a vegetarian, a high meat based diet, eating fruit, not eating fruit, food combining, etc, etc.

Now I am back to where I started, knowing what works, and my original knowledge is supported with a lot more experience.

The information I present in this book came to me and provided a great epiphany. I once again have a firm grip of the obvious.

I look back now and say, "Duh, I knew this all along."

How could I have been so stupid to believe the diet books and fitness magazines? I equate it to being stupid enough to believe when the government takes your freedoms and tells you it is for your own good and you believe them. You too will look back and say, "Duh," after reading this book.

You are about to become free!

Free from stressing over what to eat or what you just have eaten.

Free from any compulsive food disorders you may have developed over the years. Free from just eating certain foods or following a specific eating plan.

Free from feeling guilty because you had a piece of bread, or chocolate or a cheeseburger at dinner.

Free from covering up when you should be wearing a swimsuit.

Free from stressing over clothes that no longer fit.

Free from sucking down food every few hours because you believe your metabolism will slow down or your muscles will shrink if you don't.

When you no longer have to stress or worry about your weight or a specific diet, a huge weight will be lifted off your shoulders.

You are welcome in advance and yes it is ok to name your first born after me. ☺ But really I would rather you just give me cash.

Opening Thought

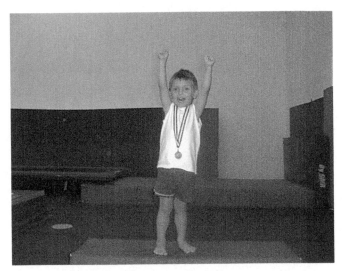

Free like a little kid!

2   Rigid Restrictions

People are free from obsessing about what, how much, and when to eat

The fact is, I admire a lot of the work that went into many of the diet books. A lot of facts and research are stated clearly. Yes, it's true that if you just eat certain foods, they will benefit your health. But if you are told you have to eat them or worse yet, you can only eat them; you will both consciously and unconsciously rebel.

There are many innovative ideas and a lot of thought put behind them. I mean, biochemically, Atkins makes great sense and different aspects of The Zone really are impressive with how hormones were studied. Ornish did a good job with his results relating to heart disease, the Protein Power Plan told how their patients responded, the list goes on and on.

If I am told, "Don't eat chocolate ever again." I want a piece of chocolate and it may consume my life and be in my thoughts until I eat that piece of chocolate.

So, first things first. Don't diet and don't put a bunch of rigid restrictions on yourself.

Here are a few questions to think about. How does it work out when the government puts restrictions on people?

The USA once restricted alcohol, how did that turn out? Bad

The USA restricts marijuana. How successful has the drug war been? Not successful at all. (The USA is a world leader per capita in putting people in jail for drug crimes).

How successful are policies in places like Amsterdam where marijuana is not restricted? Very Successful

Governments are great at putting more and more restrictions on people. They feel they should control every aspect of your life. It comes down to one person who is in power wants to actually have power over you. Throughout history these restrictions have not worked, rebellion after civil war after uprising. Just think of history class.

Are you getting the picture now? Putting rigid restrictions on people does not work.

If your diet is one that follows rigid restrictions, it will likely fail. Are you getting the picture?

And isn't your goal one that includes staying lean for the rest of your life? So your likelihood to stay on a plan that has rigid restrictions is extremely small.

You have chosen the right path with this book!

3   Does It Consume Your Life?

This eating plan is completely flexible

If you are thinking about food and your diet all the time, you are completely in the wrong mindset to get lean and stay lean.

If the diet consumes your life, you are in the wrong mindset.

Your life must be balanced for longevity. If it is not balanced, you will burn out. I have been there and done that.

I can remember my father saying, "Everything in moderation." This was a great statement, even though moderation was probably what he was worst at in life. ☺

When you are so anal about every little detail of what you are eating, it consumes your life.

I know people who are so consumed with their diet, they are thinking about their next meal while they are eating their current meal or they focus their whole week around some magical cheat meal on the weekend that consumes their thoughts and they feel horrible after eating it.

People can be successful by allowing their eating style to easily integrate without interference with other things in their life. This enables your life to be more than just dieting and what you get to eat at your next meal, which means, you can have longevity in your success.

Are there people who should be more detailed? Yes. If you have a job that is based upon your athletic performance, for instance, I would focus on choosing the foods that best fuel your body. Someone with a specific health condition would be better off choosing the foods that combat their condition and so forth.

However, most of us are in a situation that we can easily live our lifestyle and daily routine without letting our life be consumed by a special diet. This is one of the keys to your long-term success.

By making your diet a small part of your life that is so easy you don't even have to give a thought to, you are making it a part of your permanent lifestyle that guarantees your success.

Relax and enjoy these words because by the time you are done, you will feel liberated and free to enjoy food for the rest of your life while maintaining a lean and attractive body. This will be done with little to no effort.

4 My Background

If you want to read it, read it. This part does not tell the details of what to do, but it does tell you who I am and where I've been and how I came to the conclusions I am writing about. Many times you can learn by seeing what others did both right and wrong.

Don't worry, later on in this book I will be showing you the research to support what I am presenting and with each page of the book you will be feeling better and better about how easy it is for you to get lean and stay lean.

I was into weight lifting at a young age. My father, Dennis Fitzgerald, was into bodybuilding.

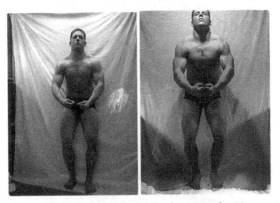

My father, Dennis Fitzgerald, as a freshman at the University of Wisconsin in 1965. Age 18.

At that time, he was one of the few football players on his college team that lifted weights. He used to tell me that the football players looked down on weight lifting at that time. Wow, how times have changed.

I started lifting weights at a young age. I bugged my dad until he wrote workouts for me. I would go into our basement in 6th grade after school and workout.

My first experience with fasting was in 7th grade during wrestling season. I weighed 127 lbs and wrestled 126 lbs. So, to make weight, I skipped dinner. That was it, simple.

With all the working out I was doing, it was paying off. I was in shape and excelling in sports. At that time in my life, I thought I was going to play pro football. Obviously it didn't work out the way I had planned.

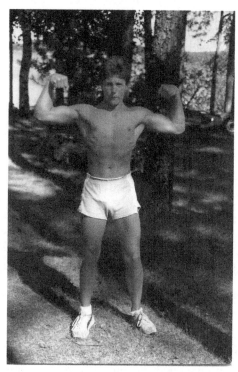

John Fitzgerald age 13

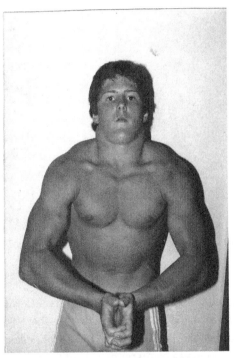

Here I am in 8th grade, age 14. I could bench press 225 lbs and
weighed 155 lbs

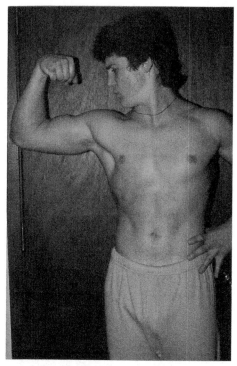

Here I am in 9th grade, age 15. I could bench press 245 lbs and weighed 165 lbs.

In 10th grade, I implemented fasting again. I will say that I didn't know what it was called or that there was even a name for it. What I did was easy; I just stopped eating after 6 pm. I was lean to begin with and got leaner.

The problem was that I played football and needed to weigh more than I did. As a senior linebacker in high school, I weighed only 183 lbs. I was lean and strong, I won weightlifter of the year for our high school, set the school record for the most tackles in a season and won All-City and All-State honors. I went to college and played football at Simpson College and lettered as a freshman where I still

12

couldn't get above 183 lbs until after the season.

I got on the football weightlifting program and started eating as much as I could at each meal in the cafeteria and my weight went up to 200 lbs. We had guys on the team who were absolutely huge; they were also taking a bunch of steroids. My knowledge of steroids was limited. The rumors that steroids shrink your balls and can make you impotent were enough to scare me to have absolutely no interest in them.

Then I realized, I wasn't going to play pro football (other than being too small and too slow I had it all going for me, lol) and I missed my girlfriend who was in school 8 hours away (we got married a couple of years later). My body was beat up from all the big hits in games and I kept getting stingers in my neck from all the hitting in football practice.

After the season ended, I went to a chiropractor, David Johnson, whose son Zach won the Masters Golf Tournament. Then I decided I would transfer schools and become a chiropractor.

Dropping my weight back down after football

After I made the decision to transfer schools and stop playing football, I remember looking in the mirror and thinking that I liked how I looked at 183 lbs better than how I looked at 200 lbs. So I did something about it. I started skipping breakfast and for lunch and dinner I would start my meal with a salad and would not eat dessert.

I was 19 yrs old and my weight dropped right back down and I was really lean again. I remember reading an article at this time, that women found men with lean athletically muscular bodies with visible abs more attractive than huge bodybuilder physiques. Really, I was lifting weights mostly to look good for girls, so it was good news to me.

I spent another 2.5 years at Kirkwood Community College getting the credits to get my Bachelors of Science degree and the credits necessary to get me into Chiropractic College. I became very interested in nutrition and started taking a bunch of chemistry classes. During this time, I decided I would get more involved in martial arts so that was my nightly training and got to a black belt level in Shotokan Karate. This was before the UFC changed the way everyone thought about martial arts.

One thing that I have noticed is that Mixed Martial Arts (cage fighting, UFC) also caused a big shift in the way people wanted to look. In the 1980's it was all about getting huge. Now it is more about getting lean and muscular. More guys want to look like a lean, athletic fighter, than a huge, steroid induced bodybuilder.

There is always going to be people that like the bodybuilder look, but the percentage is small and has shrank with the popularity of the fighter physique.

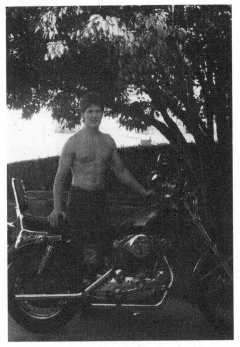

John Fitzgerald age 21

Broadcasting Football Games on the Radio

I was also asked to help broadcast on the radio high school football games and was in the booth at the Iowa Hawkeye football games. This was always a tough thing for me to accept mentally because there were a couple of guys on the Iowa team that I had played against in high school and out performed. However, they had the physical size and I didn't, so they went to the big college program and I didn't. It frustrated me for years.

One highlight, looking back now, was that I would go down on the field after the high school games and interview players. As it turned out, I was probably the first person to ever interview this quarterback from Cedar Rapids, Iowa who later became NFL great Kurt Warner.

Dad gets Cancer

Back to the story, right before I was ready to go to Chiropractic College, my dad got cancer. This is when I got heavy into nutrition. I started reading everything I could read and going to seminars about nutritional therapies. My focus was to help my dad. I changed his diet, started juicing, became a vegetarian and ate primarily raw foods. We also did quite a bit of juice fasting at that point. Remember, this was before the Internet and information was much harder to obtain. My father lost a bunch of body fat and he got healthier and recovered from his leg surgery.

Off to Chiropractic College

A couple months later, I left for Chiropractic College. At this point I was absolutely shredded (lean) and had been for quite awhile. I was obsessed with healthy nutrition and staying lean and muscular. At one point in a class for anatomy dissection lab, the instructor was going over muscles in the arm and he asked if he could show everyone muscle points on my arm. Then for the rest of the semester he would use me as a model pointing to muscles in my body because you could clearly see the separation.

In a physiology lab, we did some body fat levels with skin calipers and I registered at 3.1%. The instructor said he had worked there 10 years and never had anyone register below 7%. Who knows what I really was because how accurate are calipers anyway? The point is that I was very, very lean.

Over the next 4 years in that college, I added cooked foods back into my diet. I found it way too hard to continue doing what I was doing. My fitness completely changed again. I continued taking Karate. I stopped lifting weights. Every morning when I woke up I did 5 series of hindu bends, 2 sets of 120 pushups and 2 sets of 100 dips.

Oh yeah, I got married after my first year at this school in 1992.

Moved to South Carolina

After getting my degree, we moved. Some interesting dietary stuff went on during this period. The Zone Diet became the rage. That started to change my concept of skipping meals to having to eat frequently. I followed these concepts and found it hard to get enough protein because I was still a vegetarian at that point.

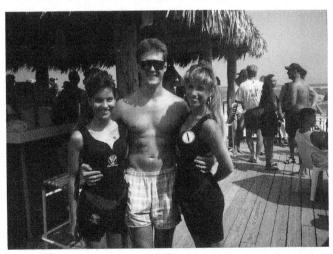

Julie Fitzgerald, John Fitzgerald age 25, Nicole. (Julie and Nicole were models for Jagermeister, thus the outfits and sticker on Julie's chest)

After a couple of years, I found a drop in my hormone levels. As it turned out, being a vegetarian wasn't the best approach. After adding meat, my levels drastically and immediately improved.

So here is where all the vegetarians discredit me, yada yada yada. Whatever dude, chill out and keep reading and this book will benefit you. I did the whole vegetarian thing for 5 years. I wouldn't classify it as being beneficial for overall health unless your vegetarian diet classification is primarily fruits and vegetables and you do eat some fish and eggs.

I added fish to my diet more regularly to follow the Zone Diet recommendations. It wasn't' until after I quit the Zone Diet that I added red meat which had the positive effect on my hormones. I found the Zone Diet too regimented and it made me feel restricted. So I quit it, but I kept the bad habits such as eating frequently. So my body fat crept up. Don't get me wrong, my scale weight only went up less than 10 lbs and I could still see my abs, but I wasn't the same level of leanness I was before.

My Practice

During this time, we opened up a clinic that was a combination of nutrition, weight loss and Chiropractic care. The local channel 2 TV station was one block from my office. A lady came in with some problems she wanted fixed and I fixed them, even after her issues had been unresolved by others.

Turns out she scheduled certain shows for channel 2 and a local radio station. She asked me to come on a 5:30 am TV show and to come on as a guest at the radio station. I did both shows and they both got a great response from callers.

So after doing a few more shows, she asked me if I would like to host a radio show. I said, "Ok" and it became a big success. I was in South Carolina and I had patients from Florida, Georgia and North Carolina coming to see me. Three other radio stations picked me up and before I knew it, I had 3000 patients.

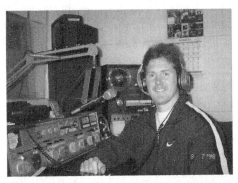

Dr. John Fitzgerald doing a radio show in 1998. It makes me laugh because I had that mustache for only a month and it is in the only picture I have at the radio station.

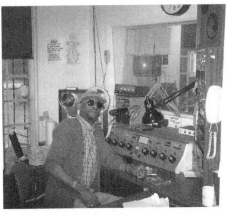

My friend, EZ Wendell in 1998, who was on the other side of the glass from me. He ran the electronics for the radio show and was a popular DJ for the station.

19

When I look back at it, there were some funny things. The first radio station that started it all was WPAL. It was the longest running all black station in the south. I am a white boy from Iowa. The south is WAY different than Iowa. I was probably the only white person that had ever been in the building, lol, and here I was hosting a show.

I can say that I was treated great at the radio station and by the black people who came into the office. They were shocked when they first saw me and discovered I am a white guy.

I was frequently invited to come lecture to large all black churches on how to fix high blood pressure and type 2 diabetes. (South Carolina leads the nation in diabetes and amputees from diabetes.) I had numerous people that came into the office who had feet cut off, had gangrene or went blind from diabetes. I can say that I helped hundreds of people normalize their blood sugars to the point their doctors were able to stop their type 2 diabetes medication. The same great results happened for blood pressure.

However, my mistake was talking about the successes and protocols on the radio. Seems like there was an accepted protocol that kept people on medications forever and I wasn't following it. So I became an enemy with the powers that be and threats were put out towards me on a regular basis. But that is a whole other story aside from this book.

Remember that this occurred before the Internet had taken off and the media could easily control what people got to hear. Clear Channel bought out WPAL as part of its national radio takeover and my show was ended. The media in the USA was quickly becoming controlled by a few sources.

Maybe my next book will be about how the government

threatens and extorts people who stand up and tell the truth. How the IRS is used to financially ruin and discredit people. How the financial systems in the USA are tied into the most corrupt systems in the world so a few sources can maintain control of your finances.

My start for your suggested reading on this topic is a book by Jake Shannon called, "Anomaly." Read it cover to cover while you are fasting.

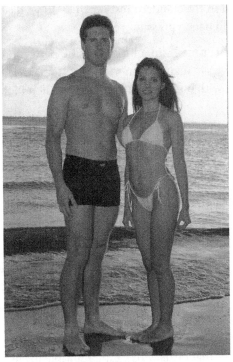

John Fitzgerald and Julie Fitzgerald both age 30, a little over a year after we had our first child Colton.

During my time in South Carolina, a football league formed that was said to be the minor league to the NFL

21

called the (NMFL) on the east coast and the team in Charleston was the Carolina Hurricanes. I don't know the details of this league other than it only lasted a few years and it was primarily guys who played college football and didn't make the NFL. Now they were playing in this league and working on advancing themselves.

I was the team doctor who was in charge of helping players improve their performance with nutrition and supplements etc. The results obtained were excellent and were measured in the standard tests such as 40 yd dash, shuttle run, 225 lb bench press for reps etc.

During this time I did a lot of athletic performance work with athletes in many different sports. It was all legal things that dealt with nutrition and optimizing their blood chemistry.

If I knew I was going to be writing a book close to 15 years later, I would have documented everything I have done, much better than I did. Thinking about it now, I would have taken way more pictures of myself and copies of blood work along the way, and I would also have taken video testimonials of patients and athletes. Oh well, shit happens and life goes on, lol.

My overall exercise after this period was mostly weightlifting sporadically. Around 1999 the Body for Life program became popular with the bodybuilding diet. This was a short-term thing I did that completely messed up my whole train of thought for several years. I talk more about this in the chapter that deals with eating multiple meals per day.

All the while I was doing these different eating programs and experimenting on myself, I was instructing patients on what to do and taking weekly body fat measurements on these same patients. So I got massive amounts of experience over several years on thousands of patients. I really got tuned in to what works and what doesn't. Many things look good in a book, but when applied, they make people feel restricted and won't be followed.

This is a clinical pearl here so memorize it

Diets fail; it's just a matter of time. The thing about fasting and skipping meals is that it's not a diet. It allows people to have freedom rather than being restricted. Unlike a diet, skipping a meal doesn't dominate your life, it completely adapts to your lifestyle.

You know when you are really good at something, yet are at the point where you are sick of it and really not that interested anymore. That's the position I was in.

After the last 3000 patients, and 4 weekly radio shows, I no longer wanted to talk to anyone again about nutrition and diet. So I sold the practice and moved to Las Vegas to do something completely different.

I decided to take my kids to Xtreme Couture to the kids grappling classes. Xtreme Couture is a premiere training facility in Las Vegas for professional fighters and and was owned by UFC Hall of Famer Randy Couture and his wife Kim Couture.

I was minding my own business, taking some grappling and kickboxing classes myself. I never spoke of what I used to do or who I was.

Then, it happened one day, I couldn't help from opening my mouth. A professional MMA fighter and wrestler with the WWE, Phil Friedman, was teaching a kettlebell class. I saw Phil was having all kinds of problems and he had a fight coming up. He was light-headed when he would standup, felt burnt out etc.

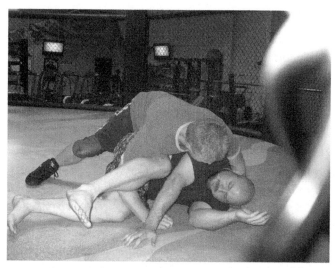

Dr. John Fitzgerald and Phil Friedman in 2008. (I like this picture because it makes me look like I am winning but in reality, Phil was teaching me a move)

I looked in Phil's eyes with a penlight and said that he had low adrenal gland output and we should do blood work and I will tell him what to do to fix it. A week later, Phil was feeling great and I was back in the game. Phil was a training partner for UFC fighter Randy Couture. Needless to say, I had bunches of MMA fighters calling me and wanting me to tell them what to do.

Then I helped Randy and Kim Couture form a supplement line and currently have regular people and professional athletes calling me from all over the country, and all over the world for that matter.

So now here I am, writing this book and counseling people on the finer points of nutrition. I promise that you will greatly benefit from the material I present and it will more importantly make your life better. Enjoy the rest of the book!

5 Metabolism

Fasting makes you more alert, makes you think clearly and puts you in-tune with your body

Short answer: Skipping meals does not slow your metabolism, as long as you lift weights to keep your muscle intact.

Metabolic rate: The basal metabolic rate is the minimum rate at which the body uses energy at complete rest. It is the minimum amount of energy needed to keep the body alive and is the largest component of an average person's daily energy expenditure. The BMR is usually expressed simply as kilocalories per day.

Muscle is metabolically more active than fat. So in general, the more muscle you have the more daily calories your body requires.

The research reviews below indicate that fasting does NOT slow metabolism. To make this easy to understand, my notes are at the beginning and are shaded.

Study: Effects of resistance vs. aerobic training combined with an 800 calorie liquid diet on lean body mass and resting metabolic rate.[1]

YOU MUST LIFT WEIGHTS while doing a low calorie diet like fasting. This preserves your muscle tissue, which keeps your metabolic rate high.

People only consumed 800 calories per day for a weight loss diet while participating in resistance exercise (weightlifting) for 12 weeks. Their lean body weight and metabolic rate were monitored. Aerobic exercise does not prevent loss of lean body weight (muscle).

Conclusion: Lifting weights (3 times per week in the study) while on a low calorie diet resulted in preservation of lean body weight (muscle) and resting metabolic rate.

Study: The cardiovascular, metabolic and hormonal changes accompanying acute starvation in men and women.[2]

Resting metabolic rate does not slow down even after 72 hours of fasting.

Resting metabolic rate was studied after 12, 36 and 72 hours of fasting in this study.

---

[1]Department of Human Performance and Applied Exercise Science, West Virginia University, Morgantown 26506, USA. J Am Coll Nutr. 1999 Apr;18(2):115-21.

[2]Department of Physiology and Pharmacology, University of Nottingham Medical School. Br J Nutr. 1994 Mar;71(3):437-47.

Study: Alternate-day fasting in nonobese subjects: effects on body weight, body composition, and energy metabolism.[3]

I found this interesting because I came to the same conclusion back around 1992. When I would fast in college I realized that I didn't like to go a whole day without eating. Eating at least 1 meal on a fasting day makes fasting much easier.

So if I fast 18 to 24 hours, it is spread out over 2 days rather than going one day without eating. For instance, I don't like going all Monday without eating, but I enjoy skipping breakfast and maybe lunch on Monday and then eating dinner on Monday.

For 22 days, people fasted every other day and *their resting metabolic rate did not slow down and their fat oxidation (burning) increased.*

Study: Restrained eating behavior and the metabolic response to dietary energy restriction in women.[4]

Metabolism was not affected.

---

[3]Pennington Biomedical Research Center, Baton Rouge, LA 70808, USA. Am J Clin Nutr. 2005 Jan;81(1):69-73.

[4]US Department of Agriculture, Agricultural Research Service, University of California, Davis, CA 95616, USA. Obes Res. 2004 Jan;12(1):141-9.

Conclusion: a 3-day low calorie diet increased the burning of fat and decreased the burning of carbs.

Study: Metabolic and behavioral compensations in response to caloric restriction: implications for the maintenance of weight loss.[5]

After 6 months, the people in the control group (the people that did nothing different than they would normally do) saw no change in their sleeping metabolic rate. *The group that did calorie restriction plus exercise also had NO change in their sleeping metabolic rate.*

The 2 other groups that either followed calorie restriction or a low calorie diet, both showed lower total daily energy expenditure.

This is another study that shows the importance of resistance (weightlifting) exercise while fasting to keep your muscle tissue intact.

---

[5]Pennington Biomedical Research Center, Baton Rouge, Louisiana, United States of America. PLoS One. 2009;4(2):e4377. Epub 2009 Feb 9.

Forty-eight overweight participants were randomized to four groups for 6-months;

Group 1 Control: energy intake at 100% of energy requirements;

Group 2 Calorie Restriction: 25% calorie restriction;

Group 3 Calorie Restriction+Exercise: 12.5% CR plus 12.5% increase in energy expenditure by structured exercise;

Group 4 Low Calorie Diet: low calorie diet (890 kcal/d) until 15% weight reduction followed by weight maintenance.

6   Snacking, Nibbling And Multiple Meals

Fat Loss the Truth doesn't require calorie counting or weighing food; and doesn't require you planning your meals or preparing your meals for days in advance

Short answer: It really doesn't matter as much as you have been told. If anything, multiple meals are worse for blood sugar than few meals.

Let's first cover the transit time for food digestion: (The answer is not simple because there are differences among people and also in the types of food eaten).

Your doctor will tell you this because we studied it so extensively in school. Here is an example of a "standard meal". These figures were in a paper from Colorado State University that took account of several studies. When you eat, this is how long it takes food to move thru your system:

- 50% of stomach contents emptied = 2.5 to 3 hours

- *Total emptying of the stomach = 4 to 5 hours*

- 50% emptying of the small intestine = 2.5 to 3 hours

- Transit through the colon = 30 to 40 hours

I really get tired of people parroting the same stuff about how you need to eat all day long. I personally don't agree with this concept for the vast majority of people. Like almost anything though, some people may love it and do well with it, I just don't think many people fall in that category.

Snacking

If there is still food in the stomach, why should a snack be eaten? It makes no sense and it teaches people to overeat. The advice of having a snack between meals is questionable, at best. The food is still in the stomach from the last meal and more food is being piled on top of it. Let your body have a break already!

There is a difference between truly being hungry and the feeling of having an empty stomach. Many people feel an empty stomach and immediately want to eat again. Many people see a time on the clock and feel they need to eat. This is all in your head from a mental habit. There is NO reason to eat again if you still have food in your stomach.

Doctors are required to take continuing education classes every year to maintain their licenses. I go to many of the cutting edge seminars where researchers and other doctors present the latest information on many topics. I find the lectures relating to anti-aging and disease prevention to be the most interesting, so I usually focus on those topics.

I was at a continuing education seminar in Las Vegas in 2010 and one lecture topic was on weight loss. Realize, that this seminar is an annual event and is known to introduce the cutting edge protocols for anti-aging and has some of the top doctors and researchers in the world giving lectures. Each speaker was giving his or her presentation on weight loss. *Every one of them spoke about Calorie Reduction. The only differences in their presentations were how to do the calorie reduction.* Some said to snack and have multiple meals, some said low carbs, some said low fat; *the ONLY similarity was Calorie Reduction!*

One lecturer who spoke was doing a low fat diet for several years, then switched to low carb diet and got much leaner in doing so. This brings up a point to keep in mind; if you aren't happy with the results you are getting, change up the food you are eating.

The most important part is lowering the calories you are consuming by skipping meals and fasting!

The next step, if you so desire, is to pay attention to what you are eating and switch it up if you want to get results that are different from what you are currently getting. Remember though, if you can't stick with it, don't bother and certainly don't stress about it.

Let me get off this tangent and back on track by talking about snacking and multiple meals.

I will take a few moments and pick on the fitness magazines. I generally don't like the magazines: Fitness magazines in general are the purveyors of huge amounts of inaccurate information. Ridiculous diets are purported, and ridiculous supplement claims are common.

Here is the thing, bodybuilding diets recommended in the magazine are extremely hard to follow and completely unnecessary. They create obsessive-compulsive disorders about food.

Let me show you a typical diet for a bodybuilder promoted in magazines:

- Meal 1: Oatmeal and egg whites

- Meal 2: Protein shake

- Meal 3: Chicken breast, rice, broccoli

- Meal 4: White fish, potatoes, green veggies or protein shake

- Meal 5: Tuna and brown rice

- Meal 6: Protein Shake

Note: it is quite common for bodybuilders to eat 7 or 8 meals per day.

My Opinion of this eating plan: I am Not a fan.

What a pain in the ass. People following this eating plan will cook their food for the whole week on Sunday night and then divide up the individual meals into Tupper ware containers.

Then they carry a backpack with all their meals for the day in it, so God forbid they miss a meal. If something happens where they do miss a meal they nearly panic. They convince themselves they are starving and they suddenly get symptoms that they create in their head like getting moody, feeling extreme hunger, and can even manifest physical symptoms like getting shaky.

One of the great marketers of this protocol to the masses was Bill Philips and his book Body for Life. Let me sum it up for you. Eat like above bodybuilding diet so you can buy a lot of his protein shakes (he was with EAS, a supplement company). Then workout with weights 3 days per week and do cardio the other 3 days per week. On your day off from exercise is your free day to eat whatever you want.

Body for Life was an ingenious book and contest with a huge winning prize. You would take before and after pictures with a newspaper to prove the picture dates. You were required to buy EAS supplements and send the receipts in with the your pictures. EAS would then pick a winner after the 12 -week contest and award a prize. This was a huge marketing success and made EAS a major player in the supplement world. What was so ingenious about this contest was that EAS required that you buy their supplements to enter the contest and recommended their protein meal replacement drinks between your food meals so it would be easier for you to eat the recommended 6 times per day.

I personally entered the contest and did this protocol. It was one of the many different eating protocols I have tried. Someone like me was not going to win it, I already had abs in my before picture but I figured it was something to motivate me to kick up my exercise program.

Here is my experience with the diet. It creates massive obsessive, compulsive behavior that lasts until you have an epiphany like I did. First off, every 3 hours I was ravenously hungry or so I thought. My days were all about my next meal. When I was eating one meal, I was thinking about the next meal. I lost my taste for food during the week because I ate the same thing over and over again. I really only looked forward to the cheat day, which my week revolved around.

If you slip up one day and have something you shouldn't, you go into the mindset of, "my whole day is ruined so I might as well just cheat the rest of the day," and in doing so you end up massively overeating because now it is a "cheat day." Then the person feels extremely guilty afterward. So they are usually miserable or guilty every day except their official cheat day and on their official cheat day they are slamming as much food as they can, because tomorrow the misery starts over again eating the same boring foods.

I have seen this scenario play out over and over with many, many patients I have counseled. I personally got leaner following this diet because I was strict with it, then afterwards I gained more body fat back than I had ever had in my life and for a while I was stuck in this train of thought even though I knew better.

Most bodybuilders walk around looking bulky and fat unless they are in a show. They cut weight for a show and then gain it back and more between shows. Each year they get a little fatter and have developed this all or nothing attitude with how they eat. It plays out something like this:

They eat a bad carb sometime during the day, now they feel they might as well consume a whole pizza, a 2-liter bottle of soda and a bag of chocolate. I really have seen it this extreme quite frequently.

Besides the whole boring meals and cheat meal problems, is the incorrect notion that they must eat every 3 hours.

They become so convinced with the bodybuilding hype that their metabolism will slow down if they don't feed their body every 3 hours; they are in a half panic if they miss a meal. This is ridiculous and completely untrue.

Their thinking becomes that they must eat more meals to increase their metabolism. Yes I know, you say the meals must be small. I say that this is true, yet hard to keep up with because you frequently come away from your meals not satisfied. I believe this goes completely against what we are genetically programmed to do, which is eat until you are satisfied and eat infrequently.

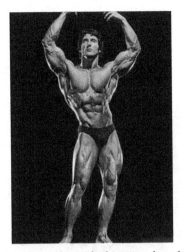

Frank Zane represents the end of an era where bodybuilding was more about aesthetics than pure size. Here he is in the late 1970's

I have a story about this. I had a trip scheduled to go to California and I decided I wanted to have a training session with Frank Zane. He was a Mr. Olympia in the late 1970's. I read his newsletters he puts out and I thought why not workout with Frank Zane once for fun.

My wife and I arrive at Frank's home in the San Diego area. His gym was the bottom floor of his house, which opened up to the back yard and some hills. Frank said, see that hill over there, that's Mexico. That was the first time I saw Mexico and it was from Frank's backyard.

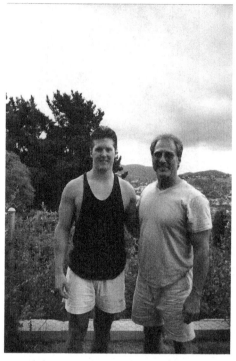

Dr. John Fitzgerald and Frank Zane 2001

So anyway, Frank had a lot of equipment and a nice setup in his home gym.

Frank was a nice guy and we spent a lot of time talking during the workout. Frank was telling me about a client that came to train with him that wanted to lose body fat. This guy apparently asked if he should eat more meals and more food to increase his metabolism. Frank laughed when he was telling this story and said he told the guy that you don't lose that fat by eating more meals and more food. I remember this very clearly because what Frank was stating was so obvious, yet people have become very confused because of fitness magazines. Frank didn't parrot back the typical stuff you read in magazines that says you must eat 6 times per day to lose body fat.

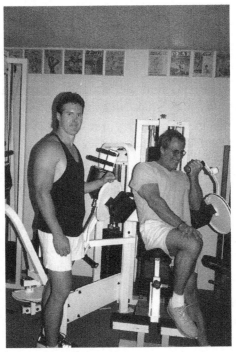

Dr. John Fitzgerald, age 31, and Frank Zane, age 59, 2001

Here is some advice from Frank's newsletter, called Building the Body, which appeared in the autumn 2004 issue. *"To get leaner I often delay eating after I get up, drinking only water with amino acids, at least one quart consumed over several hours. It might be noon before I actually eat."*

In the summer 2001 issue Frank talks about changing his diet to get leaner by his birthday. Frank says he is *"eating his last meal of the day earlier."*

(Notice that Frank, a former top-level champion fitness competitor goes longer periods without eating when he is getting lean, which means Frank spends more time in the fasted state which allows the body to burn fat as energy)

This advice is part of the Fat Loss the Truth protocol. It is one of the options that I have found patients really like and find easy to follow. You may find this simple advice completely changes how you eat as it has for many. The people that are not serious athletes do not need to take the amino acids in the morning. You will read the complete details in the Different Ways to Fast chapter.

I am sure I will get plenty of hate mail from supplement companies trying to get people to do a protein shake between each meal, so I included a few studies below. Notice that these are studies that are not done by supplement companies.

I know both regular people and bodybuilders that eat 8 times per day because they think it will help their metabolism speed up. *Once they read the studies below, it may change their minds. To make this easy to understand, my notes are at the beginning and are shaded.*

Study: Effect of the pattern of food intake on human energy metabolism.[1]

It didn't matter if the people in the study ate 2 meals per day or 7 meals per day.

[1]Department of Human Biology, University of Limburg, Maastricht, The Netherlands. Br J Nutr. 1993 Jul;70(1):103-15.

We studied the effect of meal frequency on human energy expenditure (EE) and its components. During 1 week ten male adults were fed to energy balance at two meals/day (gorging pattern) and during another week at seven meals/day (nibbling pattern).

There was no significant effect of meal frequency on 24 hour EE (energy expenditure) or ADMR (average daily metabolic rate, ADMR).

With the method used for determination, no significant effect of meal frequency on the contribution of DIT (diet-induced thermogenesis) to ADMR (average daily metabolic rate) could be demonstrated.

Study: Meal frequency and energy balance.[2]

It isn't more effective if you spread your food out into multiple meals. What matters is the amount of calories you eat.

Here is what the study said: Several epidemiological studies have observed an inverse relationship between people's habitual frequency of eating and body weight, leading to the suggestion that a 'nibbling' meal pattern may help in the avoidance of obesity.

We conclude that the *epidemiological evidence is at best very weak, and almost certainly represents an artifact (error).*

A detailed review of the possible mechanistic explanations for a metabolic advantage of nibbling meal patterns failed

---

[2]INSERM U341, Hotel Dieu de Paris, France. Br J Nutr. 1997 Apr;77 Suppl 1:S57-70.

FAT LOSS THE TRUTH

to reveal significant benefits in respect of energy expenditure.

More importantly, studies using whole-body calorimetry and doubly-labelled water to assess total 24-hour energy expenditure find no difference between nibbling and gorging.

Finally, with the exception of a single study, there is no evidence that weight loss on hypoenergetic regimens is altered by meal frequency. We conclude that any effects of meal pattern on the regulation of body weight are likely to be mediated through effects on the food intake side of the energy balance equation.

Additional note: If you are a meat head bodybuilder or some diet guru who wishes to debate me, I really don't care what you have to say unless you have actually tried what I am suggesting (skipping meals and fasting); and have counseled patients; and paid attention to the low success rates people have trying to stay on a long-term eating plan that involves eating the same thing over and over day after day 6 times per day. ☺

7   Six Meals Per Day Increases Hunger

You will find that you get a lot done when you don't have to eat every three hours

Study: The influence of higher protein intake and greater eating frequency on appetite control in overweight and obese men.[1]

This is exactly what I experienced and many patients experienced, which was increased hunger with eating multiple meals per day.

Eating less meals and more protein was shown to be satisfying.

The purpose of this study was to determine the effects of dietary protein intake and eating frequency on perceived appetite, satiety, and hormonal responses in overweight/obese men.

Thirteen men consumed diets containing:

1. normal protein (79 +/- 2 g protein/day; 14% of energy intake as protein) or

---

[1]Department of Dietetics & Nutrition, University of Kansas Medical Center, Kansas City, Kansas, USA. Obesity (Silver Spring). 2010 Sep;18(9):1725-32. Epub 2010 Mar 25.

2. higher protein (138 +/- 3 g protein/day; 25% of energy intake as protein) equally divided among three eating occasions (3-EO; every 4 hours) or

3. six eating occasions (6-EO; every 2 hours) on four separate days in randomized order.

Hunger, fullness, plasma glucose, and hormonal responses were assessed throughout 11 hours.

Independent of eating frequency, higher protein led to greater daily fullness. In contrast, higher protein led to greater daily ghrelin concentrations vs. normal protein. Protein quantity did not influence daily hunger, glucose, or insulin concentrations.

Independent of dietary protein, 6 meals per day led to lower daily fullness.

The fullness-related responses were consistently greater with higher protein intake but lower with increased eating frequency. *Collectively, these data suggest that higher protein intake promotes satiety and challenge the concept that increasing the number of meals per day enhances satiety in overweight and obese men.*

8   Carbs, Fats, Proteins

Fat Loss the Truth is simple! No counting calories, No worrying about carb, fat, protein ratios, or anything else

Short answer: Don't stress about it so much and make adjustments if needed.

This is a topic that has filled many books by itself. Should a person eat more or less of a specific macronutrient (carbs, fats, protein)? Yes it can matter, but most people should not focus on this, at least at the beginning.

I have seen that most people will drop weight faster if they eat right for themselves than they would if they just reduced calories. Yes I have a preference; I feel more people respond best to a low carb, high protein diet that is based around vegetables for the carb source.

Yet, I will make this point again, if you can't follow it, don't do it and don't stress about it. Does it really matter if you lose ½ pound per week and keep it off compared to 2 pounds per week? Whatever rate of loss that happens, it must be done in a stress free way for you to stick with it.

Also, I have found that people naturally adjust their diet to a higher percentage of healthier foods as they fast and get more in tune with when they are really hungry or not. Many people just stop eating for the sake of eating when they are not hungry and begin to choose healthier food when they do eat. This may happen to you without even realizing it.

Let's take another look at bodybuilding to see the trends that have taken place. You probably don't care about the bodybuilding, but I use some examples from bodybuilding so that you can learn why some of the diet plans that you have heard of are presenting false information.

The diet plans have changed over the years. The diet plans that were followed in the 1940's worked, yet they are much different than the diet plans today.

Have you ever looked at old muscle magazine pictures from the 50's and 60's? These guys were muscular and lean and their diets were high carb, low fat and moderate protein.

Here are a couple of pictures of Steve Reeves. He was a bodybuilder who attended chiropractic college to become a doctor then ended up becoming a highly popular movie star from that time period. He was well known for the Hercules movies of the 1950's. Steve has long been idolized as having the ideal body.

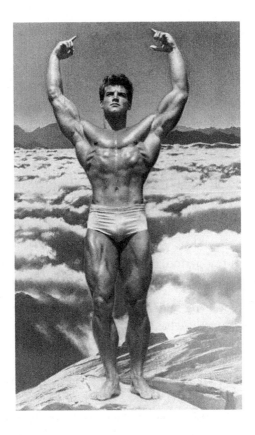

Trends have changed with time. Nowadays, bodybuilders focus on low carb, moderate fat and high protein.

My point here is this, the different ratio of carbs, fats and protein were successful in the 1950's and are completely different than what bodybuilders are currently following; yet both systems are successful today.

The same point applies to whether you are a bodybuilder or not. It also applies to men and women alike.

The bodybuilders today are much larger thanks to the advent of new and high dose steroids. As an aside point from this book is muscle gain; if you are going to put on a bunch of muscle, you are going to need to eat a bunch of food at specific times. However, the point of this book is how to become lean and stay lean. So let's stay focused on that. Maybe I will write another book specifically on how to modify things for serious athletes.

Bodybuilders both then and now have essentially gotten lean from the same thing: a calorie restricted diet. These same principles apply to everyone else also, man or woman.

You may have read that person A does a bunch of cardio while person B does no cardio or person C does wind sprints or the Tabata protocol (Periods of 100% effort followed by a rest period) once a week. *My point is that what really gets someone lean is the calorie restricted diet.*

With all that being said, I will hesitantly continue. People ask me frequently, what I prefer the most. I will say that I have seen better results with more people with the low carb and higher protein diet and I will remind you that when people are given a bunch of rules they usually don't follow them, so I am not giving you a bunch of rules. I think the best system is to start skipping meals and fasting and if you want to take it further than that you can adjust your carb, fat and protein levels.

Here are a few studies that you may find interesting: To make this easy to understand, my notes are at the beginning and are shaded.

Study: Comparison of a low-fat diet to a low-carbohydrate diet on weight loss, body composition, and risk factors for diabetes and cardiovascular disease in free-living, overweight men and women.[1]

Both eating styles got the same results in this study.

There are more conversations about the genetic predispositions to each within the doctor community. However, the main thing that should be focused on is the eating plan you can stick with. That is why I like calorie restriction from fasting and not just picking certain foods you can and can't eat.

Overweight and obese men and women (24-61 yr of age) were recruited into a randomized trial to compare the effects of a low-fat (LF) vs. a low-carbohydrate (LC) diet on weight loss. Thirty-one subjects completed all 10 weeks of the diet intervention (retention, 78%).

Subjects on the LF diet consumed an average of 17.8% of energy from fat, compared with their habitual intake of 36.4%, and had a resulting energy restriction of 2540 kJ/d.

Subjects on the LC diet consumed an average of 15.4% carbohydrate, compared with habitual intakes of about 50% carbohydrate, and had a resulting energy restriction of 3195 kJ/d.

[1]Department of Human Biology and Nutritional Sciences, University of Guelph, Guelph, N1G 2W1 Ontario, Canada. J Clin Endocrinol Metab. 2004 Jun;89(6):2717-23.

Both groups of subjects had significant weight loss over the 10 weeks of diet intervention and nearly identical improvements in body weight and fat mass.

LF subjects lost an average of 6.8 kg and had a decrease in body mass index of 2.2 kg/m2, compared with a loss of 7.0 kg and decrease in body mass index of 2.1 kg/m2 in the LC subjects.

The LF group better preserved lean body mass when compared with the LC group; however, only the LC group had a significant decrease in circulating insulin concentrations. Group results indicated that the diets were equally effective in reducing systolic blood pressure by about 10 mm Hg and diastolic pressure by 5 mm Hg.

These data suggest that energy restriction achieved by a very LC diet is equally effective as a LF diet strategy for weight loss and decreasing body fat in overweight and obese adults.

Study: Long-term effects of a very-low-carbohydrate weight loss diet compared with an isocaloric low-fat diet after 12 months.[2]

Both plans had similar weight loss. Notice that the low carb group did a better job helping with insulin resistance.

Background: Long-term weight loss and cardiometabolic effects of a very-low-carbohydrate, high-saturated-fat diet

---

[2]Preventative Health National Research Flagship, Commonwealth Scientific and Industrial Research Organization-Human Nutrition, Adelaide, SA, Australia. Am J Clin Nutr. 2009 Jul;90(1):23-32. Epub 2009 May 13.

(LC) and a high-carbohydrate, low-fat diet (LF) have not been evaluated under isocaloric conditions.

Objective: The objective was to compare an energy-controlled Low Carb diet with a Low Fat diet at 1 year.

Design: Men and women with abdominal obesity and at least one additional metabolic syndrome risk factor were randomly assigned to either an energy-restricted Low Carb diet (4%, 35%, and 61% of energy as carbohydrate, protein, and fat, respectively) or an isocaloric Low Fat diet (46%, 24%, and 30% of energy as carbohydrate, protein, and fat, respectively) for 1 year. Weight, body composition, and cardiometabolic risk markers were assessed.

Results: Sixty-nine participants completed the trial: Both groups lost similar amounts of weight and body fat. Blood pressure, fasting glucose, insulin, insulin resistance, and C-reactive protein decreased independently of diet composition. Compared with the Low Fat group, the Low Carb group had greater decreases in triglycerides, increases in HDL cholesterol and LDL cholesterol.

CONCLUSIONS: Under planned isoenergetic conditions, as expected, *both dietary patterns resulted in similar weight loss and changes in body composition. The Low Carb diet may offer clinical benefits to obese persons with insulin resistance.* However, the increase in LDL cholesterol with the LC diet suggests that this measure should be monitored.

9 Junk Food Diet / Potato Diet

With Fasting, you can still eat foods you enjoy while losing weight and maintaining weight loss and there is science to back it up

I have included these 2 diet plans to demonstrate a point and that point is this; When you reduce your calorie intake, you will lose weight.

Junk Food Diet

What happens if you eat a bunch of junk food but still eat below your required daily calorie amount? You lose weight.

In 2010, Mark Haub who is a professor of nutrition at Kansas State University, ate a bunch of junk food including Twinkies, Nutty Bars, powdered donuts, Hostess and Little Debbie snack cakes, Doritos corn chips, Oreo cookies and sugar laden cereals for two months and lost 27 pounds of body weight.

What Haub showed by eating junk food was that calorie intake is what matters most when it comes to losing weight.

Is eating junk food healthier for your body than eating vegetables? Of course not. We are back to common sense here; vegetables have a lot of nutrients in them that have a healthy and protective effect on the body.

However, if you drop your calories, you can lose weight by eating vegetables, fruit, meat and yes, junk food.

Sometimes in life people jump over dollar bills to pick up pennies. They get so involved with the details that they completely miss the big point. *The big point here or the "dollar bill" with weight loss is that you have to eat fewer calories to lose weight.*

The "pennies" (very minor details) here are very small issues like this for instance; can I eat junk food, or fruit, or meat etc.

If someone asks me these questions I know they haven't gotten it yet; the idea has not clicked for them, so I then start to explain it over again in a slightly different way. I will explain to them that they must cut calories and that is what is the most important detail. That is what this book is doing, explaining the point that lowering calories means losing body fat over and over again with many examples and lots of research.

Trust me, your doctor is likely very busy seeing patients and cannot take time to explain this point over and over again; so this book is doing the repeated explanations for your doctor. I present the same point over and over in a slightly different way so it makes sense to you.

Funny thing is that if you were 10 years old it would be very easy to explain, but many people have so much wrong information in their heads they confuse a very simple fact.

Here it is again as professor Haub pointed out on himself, cutting calories causes you to lose weight and we feel that the easiest way to cut calories is by skipping meals and fasting while eating the foods you enjoy when you do eat.

Ok, let's get back to Haub. He used to eat 2600 calories per day and cut to 1800 calories per day.

His body mass index went from 28.8, considered overweight, to 24.9, which is normal. He now weighs 174 pounds.

His HDL good cholesterol increased 20%.

His LDL bad cholesterol lowered 20%.

His triglycerides lowered 39%, which is very good.

His body fat went from 33.4% to 24.9%.

When it was all said and done, 2/3 of his calorie intake came from junk food.

Another thing I will point out is that obesity causes many health problems; diabetes, high blood pressure, heart problems for instance. Obesity is now a leading cause of premature, preventable death.

So if it takes eating junk food to lose weight, what is the problem with that? It goes back to what I say and what your doctor will tell you, whatever you enjoy and can stick to, is what you should be doing.

When people start following the protocols of skipping meals in Fat Loss the Truth, they typically start to naturally choose healthier foods without even paying attention to it. It just becomes a natural thing.

So what if you eat 65% junk food at the beginning and end up eating 25% junk food after a few months. If this is what makes you happy and helps you to get lean and stay lean, go for it.

One time I went 8 weeks with eating perfectly and I mean perfectly. Not even one piece of pizza, which is my favorite food. What ended it was, I went to a party and stared and stressed about the cake and pizza and Chik-fil-a nugget platter. So I finally gave in and ate and the 8 weeks of being perfect ended. For 8 weeks I was stressed and thought about food all the time. This is no way to live.

My body fat started to creep up a bit after I followed an

eating plan that required me to eat 6 times per day. For a few years I abandoned common sense and had a planned cheat day and multiple meals per day. Soon, I could no longer refrain myself to keep 1 cheat day per week and it went to multiple "cheat days" per week. I do not believe in these scheduled cheat days and constantly eating meals. This was a big mistake that I rectified by going back to the protocols in Fat Loss the Truth.

I will say that I have leaned up just as good as I did eating perfectly for 8 weeks when I ate all the foods I wanted and whatever I was hungry for. I did not stress over food, nor was food constantly on my mind. What did I do you ask? I followed the protocols in this book. I usually ate dinner around 6 pm and didn't eat again until noon the next day and a couple days a week I would skip the meal at noon and only eat dinner that day. It is extremely simple and puts you in a state of freedom when it comes to food.

The Potato Diet

Chris Voigt, the head of the Washington State Potato Commission, went on a 60-day diet where all he ate was potatoes.

Voigt's job is to promote potatoes, which have recently received a lot of bad publicity from the various low carb diets. As you probably already know, potatoes are primarily carbs and therefore low carb diets recommend avoiding potatoes.

So he wanted to prove a point that potatoes are a healthy food. By the way, potatoes are considered a "starchy" vegetable and contain a significant amount of fiber and vitamin C among other micronutrients.

Voigt ate 20 potatoes per day, which still created a calorie deficiency for him. So what happened you ask? He lost 21 pounds in the 2 months he ate only potatoes. He did have his cholesterol level checked and it dropped by 67 points also.

This is yet another example that cutting calories causes weight loss. Any person will find that skipping some meals and fasting is much, much easier than only eating potatoes for 60 days.

10 The "Ripped" books

The cycle of deprivation, guilt and binging will be ended with fasting. You will never feel like a cheater again

A quick overview: when getting lean, diet is what counts rather than doing hours of cardio.

The "Ripped" books are a series of books written by lawyer and fitness writer Clarence Bass. At the time of writing this book, Clarence is 73 years old and still ripped. His stuff is impressive because he has documented himself with pictures and journals keeping track of what he ate and how he exercised for nearly 60 years, which is a phenomenal amount of information.

Do a web search on Clarence Bass and look at his pictures over the years. This isn't a guy that would periodically get lean for a competition. This is a guy who walked around ripped (very lean) for his entire adult life.

What I learned from Clarence is that getting ripped is primarily about diet and not so much about doing cardio. In one of his books he details how he dropped his body fat % to 2.4% when he was over the age of 40.

Clarence's diet goes against the trend in bodybuilding of eating a high protein, low carb diet, which is another example of what the main theme of this book is about. *Cutting your calories is how you get lean and the easiest way to cut calories is outlined in the chapter "Different ways to Fast".*

Clarence is a machine! He is a true outlier (A term for someone outside of the norm). I look at him with amazement for what he has been able to accomplish. Very few people would ever follow the eating plan that he has been able to follow. Clarence eats the same thing day after day and eats a bunch of meals that most people simply will not eat. If you do exactly what he does, it works, but it is another example of putting together a program that is rigidly restrictive that takes a rare person such as Clarence to actually follow.

According to his book "Challenge Yourself", Clarence eats a breakfast everyday of cooked grains like kamut, amaranth and oat groats. Adds some skim milk and black beans, a little fruit like peaches and apple, some sesame seeds and flax seeds and then a little protein powder in the mix. This is all eaten in a bowl mixed together.

Lunch is a veggie burger with whole grain bread and some yogurt with some fruit and flax seeds mixed in.

Dinner is a stew that he puts in mixed veggies, yogurt, beans, and a can of fish like salmon or sardines. He eats a couple of pieces of whole grain bread with his stew.

I have tried eating exactly the way Clarence does and failed miserably. Like I say, I admire what Clarence has done and his incredible ability to stay with it year after year, but I have no desire to eat these foods and I didn't have any patients that lasted more than a week doing this. Most wouldn't even start it to begin with when I showed them what I wanted them to eat...lol

His books include his fitness routines, and what he has learned over the years. I will sum it up:

Lift weights and make it challenging

Rotate your workouts

Walk for an hour a day (not cardio, just a walk to stay active)

Clarence does a high intensity interval cardio session like sprints 1 time per week. He likes a rowing machine and a Schwinn Airdyne also.

He gives some good insights for training in his book Challenge Yourself. Those of you who have trained for many years can relate to needing to find ways to stay inspired and wanting the most results from the least amount of workouts which Clarence covers.

Conclusion

I added this chapter on Clarence Bass because he did not follow the typical low carb diets that are popular at the time of writing this book. Clarence stays lean all year around and has done so for his adult life.

This is an example, which shows that Clarence got lean primarily from calorie restriction, not some magical ratio of protein to carbs to fat.

I have not followed this point closely, but Clarence's wife has been following the same diet plan and has reaped the physical health benefits just like Clarence has.

His main activity has always been weightlifting and Clarence has come to the conclusion that it should be done intensely once per week.

Personally I go through vastly different periods of Motivation when it comes to exercise. Right now, I really like Clarence's ideas of one weightlifting session per week and one intense cardio session and walking on the other days. I do the walking when I am on the phone during the business day and stand the rest of the business day.

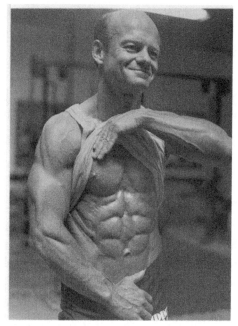

Clarence Bass age 43

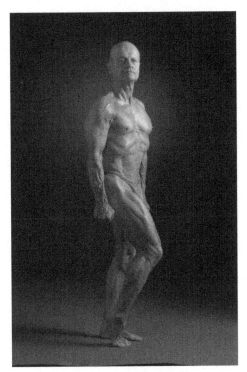

Clarence Bass age 70

11   Decreasing Calories Is What Is Important

After a person gets used to fasting, they will never be "starving" again. You will learn what it is like to be truly hungry and ignore the false hunger

Ok, this is incredibly simple, many different diets, virtually any diet for that matter, work as long as there is a decrease in a person's caloric intake.

What is important is that you realize that the best diet (eating plan) for YOU is one that you LIKE, will easily STAY ON and decreases your caloric intake.

So wouldn't the best solution be to not go on a diet at all, yet to do something that decreases calories? That is what this book explains to you how to do.

The thing is, I don't even consider skipping meals and fasting a diet. You do not have restrictions and can eat what you want. The strategies in Fat Loss the Truth work because during the times of fasting, you are not eating calories, which results in weight loss through calorie restriction.

This is a perfect way to lose fat and to maintain fat loss and stay lean.

There are 2 phases that your body can be in when it comes to eating and not eating. Both states are normal. How much time you spend in each state can make all the difference in the world with fat loss *and your overall health. Here are the universally accepted terms:*

1. Fasting – burning stored calories while not eating

2. Fed – using and storing calories from eating

To eliminate confusion, you are still in the Fed state for several hours after you eat. There is more info about how long it actually takes for a meal to digest in the "Snacking, Nibbling and Multiple Meals" chapter.

This book will show you how easy it is to spend more time in the Fasting phase. This is so easy and simple to do that you may wonder why you were never explained this in school. (Hopefully, our society has advanced to the point where this book is given out in schools and colleges).

Imagine how this simple information can turn around the trend of obesity in our society. As easy as the obesity epidemic started, it can also easily end with the information in this book. You see, in life, the magic, the solution, is usually in the simplicity.

There are such bad misconceptions about fat loss. As I am writing this, my niece called and asked what protein shake she should get. I asked why and she said she wanted to lose some fat so thought she would drink a protein shake between meals. I quickly informed her that strategy would make her gain weight, not lose weight. You don't lose weight by adding calories to your diet. You are starting to understand this right?

One of the reasons I am writing this book, besides wanting to get filthy rich and drive a Ferrari, ☺ is that I get sick of saying the same thing over and over when counseling patients and athletes. So I figure I can have them read the book and it will save me a bunch of time as well as giving society an epiphany that losing weight is really a simple mind shift about either being Fed or Fasting.

Here are a couple studies showing that the most important thing about weight loss is calorie restriction: To make this easy to understand, my notes are at the beginning and are shaded.

Study: Short term effects of energy restriction and dietary fat sub-type on weight loss and disease risk factors.[1]

A low calorie diet had the most positive effect on weight loss.

Decreasing energy intake relative to energy expenditure is the indisputable tenet of weight loss. In addition to caloric restriction modification of the type of dietary fat may provide further benefits. The aim of the present study was to examine the effect of energy restriction alone and with dietary fat modification on weight loss and adiposity, as well as on risk factors for obesity related disease.

Methods and Results: One-hundred and fifty overweight men and women were randomized into a 3 month controlled trial with four low fat (30% energy) dietary arms:

1. isocaloric (LF)
2. isocaloric with 10% polyunsaturated fatty acids (LF-PUFA)
3. low calorie (LF-LC) (-2MJ)
4. low calorie with 10% PUFA (LF-PUFA-LC).

[1]Smart Foods Centre, University of Wollongong, Wollongong, NSW 2522, Australia. Nutr Metab Cardiovasc Dis. 2010 Jun;20(5):317-25. Epub 2009 Jun 30.

Primary outcomes were changes in body weight and body fat and secondary outcomes were changes in fasting levels of leptin, insulin, glucose, lipids and erythrocyte fatty acids.

Changes in dietary intake were assessed using 3 day food records. One-hundred and twenty-two participants entered the study and 95 completed the study. All groups lost weight and body fat, but the *Low Calorie (LC) groups lost more weight.* All groups reduced total cholesterol levels, but the LC and PUFA groups were better at reducing triacylglycerol levels.

Conclusion: Energy restriction has the most potent effect on weight loss and lipids, but fat modification is also beneficial when energy restriction is more modest.

Study: Effect of energy-reduced diets high in dairy products and fiber on weight loss in obese adults.[2]

Once again, this study showed that the most important thing with weight loss is lowering how many calories are eaten.

The effects on weight loss and body fat of a diet high in dairy and fiber and low in glycemic index were compared with a standard diet.

90 obese subjects were recruited into a randomized trial of three diets designed to provide a calorie deficit of 500 calories/day over a 48-week period. The study compared a moderate (not low)-calcium diet with a high-calcium diet.

---

[2]Mayo Clinic Graduate School of Medicine, Division of Preventive and Occupational Medicine, Rochester, MN 55905, USA. Thompson. Obes Res. 2005 Aug;13(8):1344-53.

Results: Seventy-two subjects completed the study. Significant weight and fat loss occurred with all three diets.

A diet with 1400 mg of calcium did not result in greater weight or fat loss than a diet with 800 mg of calcium.

A diet with 1400 mg of calcium, increased fiber content, and fewer high-glycemic index foods did not result in greater weight or fat loss than the standard diet with 800 mg of calcium.

Lipid profile, high-sensitivity C-reactive protein, leptin, fasting glucose, and insulin improved significantly, but there were no significant differences between the experimental diets and the control diet.

Discussion: We found no evidence that diets higher than 800 mg of calcium in dairy products or higher in fiber and lower in glycemic index enhance weight reduction beyond what is seen with calorie restriction alone.

12   Fasting Gets Lasting Results

Many people start fasting once they learn how easy weight loss can be

Not only is fasting the easiest method for weight loss, the research says it is the most effective.

Study: Fasting - the ultimate diet?[1]

Short term fasting was more effective at weight loss than low calorie diets and very low calorie diets.

After 1 year, the people who utilized fasting maintained their weight loss; and the people who utilized the low calorie diets and very low calorie diets gained all the weight back.

Adult humans often undertake acute fasts for cosmetic, religious or medical reasons. For example, an estimated 14% of US adults have reported using fasting as a means to control body weight and this approach has long been advocated as an intermittent treatment for gross refractory obesity.

There are unique historical data sets on extreme forms of food restriction that give insight into the consequences of starvation or semi-starvation in previously healthy, but usually non-obese subjects. These include documented

---

[1]Rowett Research Institute, Aberdeen, UK. A. Obes Rev. 2007 May;8(3):211-22.

medical reports on victims of hunger strike, famine and prisoners of war.

Such data provide a detailed account on how the body adapts to prolonged starvation. It has previously been shown that fasting for the biblical period of 40 days and 40 nights is well within the overall physiological capabilities of a healthy adult. However, the specific effects on the human body and mind are less clearly documented, either in the short term (hours) or in the longer term (days).

This review asks the following three questions, pertinent to any weight-loss therapy, (i) how effective is the regime in achieving weight loss, (ii) what impact does it have on psychology? and finally, (iii) does it work long-term?

13   Different Ways to Fast – Immediate Start Instructions

Fasting and skipping meals gets easier and easier as time goes on. This is a phenomenon that truly puts you in tune with your body

1. Daily fasting

2. Fasting 1-3 times per week

3. Combination of both

I will say this. I have done all 3 methods and counseled people in all 3 methods. I suggest that you do all 3 and see what you like the best, what is the easiest to follow and what gives you the best results.

I have also experimented around with other strategies that I have found were not as effective and or not as easy to follow, so I am not confusing you by listing them here.

It is NOT recommended to eat snacks. There is no need to eat between meals.

1. Daily Fasting

Daily fasting is what I started doing in 10th grade when I decided not to eat after 6pm. I saw results just skipping the snack I used to eat after dinner.

I would suggest starting with something like this:

Eat dinner at 6 or 7 or 8 pm. (I like around 6 pm) and then don't eat again until lunch the next day at approximately noon where you will eat a reasonable lunch and a reasonable dinner at 6 or 7 or 8 pm.

This is easy to do and I usually tell people to go a minimum of 16 hours without eating. *I personally like fasting approximately 18 hrs daily, which is 6pm until noon the next day.*

You basically skip breakfast and then eat a reasonable lunch and a reasonable dinner.

In counseling others for fat loss, I think that this is a very easy way to start.

An example of when to eat every day:

(Skip Breakfast)   Eat Lunch   Eat Dinner

Repeat this each day. Eat dinner 6 hours or less after lunch. Then eat lunch the next day 18 hours after dinner. You adjust the hours to your schedule.

2. Fasting 1-3 times per week

Each fast is generally 22 to 24 hours.

This is based on eating 3 meals per day. So you will generally skip 2 meals during the fasting day.

For instance, say you eat dinner tonight at 6 pm and then you eat again tomorrow at 6 pm, you will have fasted 24 hours. Simple and easy.

It doesn't have to be 6 pm. You can start at 1 pm, right after lunch and not eat again until 1 pm the next day. Whatever works for you is ok. Play around with it. The plan is to skip 2 meals and go 22 to 24 hours without eating.

I played around with fasting when I was in college in the early 1990's and sometimes fasted for 3 days. If your goal is maintaining your metabolism and losing body fat, I can tell you that the difficulty goes up and the benefits go down after 24 hours of not eating as you will read in this book.

You may find as others have that around 22 hours takes little effort or thought. For instance, eat a reasonable dinner at 6 pm and don't eat again until 4 pm the next day. (I like to have an early dinner the next day and then not eat again until noon the following day) Easy peasy lemon squeezy.

An example of a 24 hour fast:

Day 1
Eat Breakfast at 8am Eat Lunch at 12pm Eat Dinner at 6pm

Day 2
(Skip Breakfast) (Skip Lunch)   Eat Dinner at 6pm

Day 3
Eat Breakfast   Eat Lunch   Eat Dinner

Many people like to do this strategy 1 - 3 times per week.

75

When I first read about fasting, the book I read said to fast for 1 day so I would go one waking day without eating, which usually amounted to 36 hours. Then I read in another place that they recommended 24 hours. I greatly prefer 24 hours to 36 hours because I think it is way easier to fast when you have at least 1 meal in a waking day. I enjoy fasting for 24 hours; yet do not look forward to 36 hours, which requires me to skip a waking day without eating. I do what I enjoy, which is usually 22 to 24 hours without eating.

3. Combination of Both

This is how I found fasting to work the best if you want to speed up the weight loss.

Do the daily fast as described above where you fast for 16 to 18 hours by skipping breakfast.

Then once or twice per week add a little longer fast of 22 to 24 hours.

This is simple to do. Let's say your routine is that you stop eating at 6 pm every night and eat lunch the next day at noon. You are already used to fasting 18 hours per day. Now, once or twice a week, you will skip that noon meal and wait until dinner to eat.

This is great to do on a day that you know you will be busy. Again, don't force yourself to have a rigid day that you have to do it on. One week it may be on Monday and the next week Wednesday. It doesn't matter.

This is very effective when you want to speed up the weight loss.

Day 1		
(Skip Breakfast)	Eat Lunch	Eat Dinner

Day 2		
(Skip Breakfast)	(Skip Lunch)	Eat Dinner

Day 3		
(Skip Breakfast)	Eat Lunch	Eat Dinner

Realize that doing something that you stick with over time is the key. Do what is easy and what you enjoy.

Remember this; decreasing calories is what is important and it doesn't have to be the same everyday. Think of how you are decreasing calories over a longer period of time like a week or month.

Maybe you eat a little too much on one day and then the next day you skip 2 meals and only eat dinner. So for those 2 days you are equal or lower than the calories your metabolism needs. Skip another couple of meals a few days later and you are burning more body fat and are losing weight overall for the week. You will notice that fasting becomes a positive event that is easily used to lose and then maintain your weight.

So why do I like the time periods of 18 hours for daily fasting and 24 hours for fasting 1-3 times per week?

Originally I liked these times because I thought they were the easiest to follow.

Then I read the study below and 18 to 24 hours happened to be the sweet spot for fasting.

Just like almost anything in life, there is a point that gets most of your results with the minimum effort and 18 to 24 hours is the spot for fasting.

I have gone three waking days without eating, but I never liked doing it. I felt the difficulty level rose dramatically when all along the majority of the results I was receiving was occurring within the first 24 hours (which I enjoy doing).

It reminds me of the 80/20 rule. In 1906, an Italian named Vilfredo Pareto created a mathematical formula to describe wealth. He observed that 20% of the people owned 80% of the wealth. Other people started applying the principle to different areas of study. With project managers, the first 10% and last 10% (total 20% of the work) takes up 80% of your time. With sales, 20% of your staff will provide 80% of your production.

Many people have said that 20% of your efforts get 80% of the results. Therefore the value in this rule is to focus on the 20% that matters or as other people like to say is to focus 80% of your time and energy on the most important 20%.

Here is a study that shows with fat loss, the first 24 hours of fasting gives you the most results: To make this easy to understand, my notes are at the beginning and are shaded.

Study: Progressive alterations in lipid and glucose metabolism during short-term fasting in young adult men.[1]

The sweet spot for fasting occurs between 18 and 24 hours. Fasting for 18 to 24 hours is easy and most of the beneficial results take place during this time such as lowering insulin levels so fat can be burned as energy.

Stable isotope tracers and indirect calorimetry were used to evaluate the progressive alterations in lipid and glucose metabolism after 12, 18, 24, 30, 42, 54, and 72 hours of fasting in six healthy male volunteers.

Of the total increase in lipid (fat) rate of change, 60% occurred between 12 and 24 hours of fasting; the greatest interval change occurred between 18 and 24 hours of fasting.

Glucose rate of appearance and plasma concentration decreased by approximately 25% between 12 hours and 72 hours of fasting, but no statistically significant changes occurred between 18 and 24 hours of fasting.

Plasma insulin decreased by approximately 50% between 12 hours and 72 hours of fasting. *Of the total decline in plasma insulin, 70% occurred within the first 24 hours of fasting.*

These results demonstrate that the mobilization of adipose tissue triglycerides increases markedly between 18 and 24 hours of fasting in young adult men.

---

[1]Department of Internal Medicine, University of Texas Medical Branch, Galveston 77555. Am J Physiol. 1993 Nov;265(5 Pt 1):E801-6.

14   How To Eat

Any person can do this and so can you. It really is this easy

Do I have a preference on how to eat?

Yes.

Do I think most people will follow it?

No.

Do I think you should stress yourself over following it?

No.

So what is it? The eating strategy that I have seen help the professional athletes and regular patients of mine is this: focus on a variety of fruits, vegetables, wild caught fish, grass-fed meat, poultry and nuts. There are many books that go into detail and document all the research on eating like this. There are big health benefits if you can follow this strategy.

So my recommendation is this, Eat Reasonable in a way where you are happy to skip meals.

What does that mean? There isn't a direct definition of this but I will make it simple. KISS method (Keep it simple stupid)

Eat a reasonable sized meal when you eat. Do not overfeed yourself.

You will NOT eat more right after the fast or right before the fast, eat a reasonable sized meal just as you would at other times.

Can you fast and still gain weight? Yes of course you can.

But that is why you eat reasonably sized meals. Interestingly enough, this was not a typical problem I have seen with patients. People know this without having to harp on it.

Remember my statement earlier about having a firm grip of the obvious.

Well isn't it obvious that if you choose to eat more fruits and vegetables, that will be healthier than eating French fries?

I have to laugh about this for a minute. I had a guy actually debate me on this once over dinner. We debated between broccoli and French fries. Everyone just listened in amazement at the ridiculous stuff coming out of his mouth and to top it off he was at least 100 lbs overweight and diabetic with raging uncontrolled blood sugar.

A friend, who was with me at the dinner, and I could not stop laughing after the dinner at how ridiculous this actually was. I mean come on already, this is common sense stuff. Don't make the obvious confusing. Broccoli has more health benefits than French fries...duh!

However, if you want pizza, eat it and enjoy it because you are still creating a calorie deficiency with your fasting and you will still achieve your goals. The most important part is the fasting part and not stuffing yourself before or after the fast.

I find that people start naturally choosing healthier foods without really even thinking about it once they start fasting. It is definitely a phenomenon that happens with little thought and happens to most people.

Maybe their stomachs shrink; maybe their unconscious mind is picking healthier food. Once you start eating this way you may find that you too, start choosing healthier food between fasts also.

15   What Can I Drink During Fasting Hours?

Water – Yes   This should be what you usually drink.

Tea – Yes   I like to drink a big glass everyday. Tea has a lot of health benefits, especially green tea.

Coffee - Yes   I seriously love coffee. I didn't even try coffee until I was 30 yrs old. Ever since I was a little kid, all I ever saw my hunched over grandma drinking was coffee all day long so I associated coffee with old people.

Then my wife introduced me to the dark side (which is straight black coffee) and I was hooked. ☺

I would rather drink coffee than alcohol hands down. I guess I like stimulants rather than depressants.

Have too much coffee in the morning and it turns your stomach and makes you feel like you need food instantly.

Have the right amount of coffee and it perks you right up.

Drink it black. It's really good sprinkling cinnamon in it.

You don't add stuff like sweeteners, sugar, milk, cream etc during fasting hours.

I like to drink coffee and water at the same time, sip for sip. I feel it tastes better with each drink and I feel better doing it that way.

Sodas – No   I feel sodas are extremely harmful to your biochemistry. Sodas are a conglomeration of chemicals that make your body acidic. In your spare time do a web search and learn how damaging it is when you are acidic.

Regular sodas are an obvious No because of the calories.

Diet sodas – are a No also.

Have you ever noticed that obese people and people with a lot of health problems drink diet sodas as their regular fluid they intake? It used to drive me crazy how ignorant and brainwashed people are. Here is a typical example that would come into my office.

A diabetic that has had a foot removed comes into my office drinking a diet soda and proceeds to show me the gangrene on his other foot. I told him the first thing he must do is dump out that soda on his way to the hospital. He told me that it is "ok" because it is a diet soda.

I explain how diabetes is an acidic condition and that diet soda is highly acidic and then I would go into how it affects the hunger centers of the brain etc. Then after time, my standard reply became, do not come back to me until you put together information to share with me about how diet soda makes diabetes worse. It was funny because people came back happy to share with me all the negative information they had researched.

Why the hell do fitness trainers and bodybuilders drink diet sodas all day long when there are so many health risks associated with them? Apparently they think it is ok because diet sodas claim to have 0 or reduced calories.

So I have a pro MMA fighter who is complaining of bad endurance. Of course he used to be a bodybuilder and is still drinking 6 diet sodas per day. I do blood work on him and his CO_2 level is reduced. Here is a little insight; CO_2 acts like a buffer system in your blood. If the level drops, it means you are using more buffer to neutralize acid. In other words, his low CO2 level means he was over acidic. Over acidic equals low endurance.

This pro fighter made himself acidic sucking down diet sodas all day long which caused his endurance to tank. I explained what happened and told him to stop the diet sodas, switch to green tea which is alkaline, add 2 green drinks (powdered vegetables mixed in water or a protein shake) per day and minerals for alkalinity and this will fix it. His endurance drastically improved.

Fruit juice – No   It has a bunch of calories

Any other drink with calories that I haven't listed – No

Can I add sugar or calories to my drinks? – No

16   Calorie Math For Fasting

Fat Loss the Truth fits perfect with your job and lifestyle plus you will never have to say you are on a diet again

Calorie counting is effective but is tedious work that most people stop doing after a short period of time.

Let's do some basic math here to discover how simple and effective fasting is:

3 meals per day × 7 days per week = 21 meals per week

I wonder what would happen if you ate 19 or even 17 meals per week instead of 21? A person would, you know, lose weight.

Let's say you fast for 24 hours. For instance, you eat lunch on Monday at noon and then decide to fast for the next 24 hours. Then you skip dinner on Monday and breakfast on Tuesday. (You will have skipped 2 meals). Then you resume normal eating for lunch at noon on Tuesday.

Monday
Eat Breakfast   Eat Lunch   (skip it)

Tuesday
(skip it)   Eat Lunch   Eat Dinner

Wednesday
Eat Breakfast   Eat Lunch   Eat Dinner

If you fasted one 24- hour period, you will have skipped 2 meals, which is 9.5% of your weekly food intake.

If you fasted two 24- hour periods, you will have skipped 4 meals, which is 19% of your weekly food intake.

Now let's break these figures down to calories.

Eating 700 calories per meal would yield 2100 calories per day and 14,700 calories per week.

If you fasted one 24- hour period, you will have skipped 2 meals, which is 1400 calories.

If you fasted two 24- hour periods, you will have skipped 4 meals, which is 2800 calories. If you kept all your other days the same, this will be equivalent to reducing 400 calories per day.

These are significant calorie decreases that will cause your body to lose fat. Think about how nice it is to lose body fat without going on a diet and just simply incorporating skipping meals into your routine.

Counting calories is something that is effective if someone actually sticks with it. When I was a student, I had to record everything I ate for a period of time. I was recording every ingredient I ate, and the exact amount. If my dinner had 20 ingredients, this recording process took a bunch of time. This was before the internet and before everyone had computers so I did this all by hand. Now it is easier with internet programs, but it is still a lot of work.

With a busy lifestyle, I don't see many people that will actually record all their calories. How most people find calorie counting useful is to do it for a short period of time to get an idea of how much they are actually consuming in a day and then make adjustments if necessary. In other words, it is a tool that provides you with awareness.

17   Don't Fast If

This question always comes up. Who should NOT fast?

1. Children

2. Pregnant women…Pregnant men are ok ☺

3. People with any medical conditions. (Check with your doctor first)

4. People with eating disorders such as anorexia.

When in doubt, check with your doctor if they gave you this book. If not, give a copy to your doctor, then ask them questions AFTER they read this book.

18 Fasting Gets Easier By The Week

Everyday that you complete a fasting period brings a sense of victory. You really feel good about yourself and this feeling continues to grow

Most diets get harder and harder to follow because they are restrictive, and after time your temptations will give in to those natural urges.

This is completely the opposite with fasting, which gets easier because your mind and body starts to adapt and form new habits that are actually easy to follow.

Unlike other eating styles or diet plans, "Fat Loss the Truth" gets easier each week!

The first few times a meal is skipped, you are not quite sure what to think. You are altering old habits and getting used to something different.

I wonder if you have ever thought that something would be difficult, and while you were doing it, it wasn't difficult, but you kept saying to yourself, "This should be getting hard any moment", yet it never did get hard.

Afterwards, you questioned yourself, "Is that it? Isn't this supposed to be hard?" and yet, it remained relatively easily to do.

This is a typical reaction. "I can't believe it is this easy. I really feel better doing this."

While you're fasting and realizing how easy it is, you can rest assured that fasting is the easiest approach to losing fat and then maintaining your weight.

19 You're Not Really Hungry

Fasting allows you to learn when you are hungry and when it is just mental. Fasting exposes your habits. A person can understand if they're eating because of a habit or actual hunger

Let's start by covering the obvious once again.

Remember what was covered earlier in this book. Many times, the stomach is not empty until 5 hours after you eat a meal and there is certainly no reason to be hungry if you still have food in your stomach.

Take that a step further, and remember that is takes another 3 hours after the food leaves the stomach for just 50% of the food to empty out of the small intestine. We are talking about an extended period of time that it takes your meal to digest. We call this being in the Fed state.

Eating a little bit just makes you hungry

I saw a recommendation once where a nutritionist made a recommendation to eat 6 almonds as a snack.

I just don't think we are programmed to eat small snacks. I instantly think what my cousin said at one meal when we were talking "That's just enough to piss you off", and he is right. Eating 6 almonds is just enough to piss me off.

Listen, I am not arguing if "The Zone" or "Body for Life" or any other diet book really works or not. I am arguing that they are way too hard to stick to. Your life revolves around the diet and you become obsessed with it and this is the problem.

In World War II the Allied Forces were worried about German submarines, so they went to a scientist to solve the problem. The scientist came back with findings, which said that to get rid of the submarines, all that has to be done is to raise the temperature of the oceans. Well, yes that would work but how do we go about raising the temperature of the oceans? This is similar with the diet books, they tell you what works, but they do it with unrealistic recommendations.

Eating a small snack when you are truly hungry isn't going to satisfy you and eating a snack when you still have food in your stomach is conditioning yourself to eat when you are not truly hungry.

That leads me to discuss conditioning yourself to form destructive habits, like eating when you still have food in your stomach.

It's all in your head

Ivan Pavlov was a scientist who won the Nobel Prize in 1904. His description on how animals and humans can be trained to respond in a certain way to a certain stimulus, paved the way for a new method of studying behavior.

We have all heard the story about Pavlov's dogs. If you haven't, here is the brief summary. Pavlov analyzed saliva response in dogs under different conditions. Pavlov noticed that the dogs started to salivate before the food reached their mouths. So then Pavlov started to study what he called this "psychic secretion."

The dogs drooled with no food in sight because the dogs were reacting to lab coats. Whenever the dogs were served food, the people who served the food were wearing lab coats. The dogs reacted as if food was on its way whenever they saw a lab coat.

He later used striking a bell to associate the dogs with food.

I think people create associations the same way and many times it is something as simple as the time on a clock. For instance, a person sees 7:30 AM on the clock and reacts as if it's time to eat breakfast or they see 3 pm and feel that they need a snack. It's merely a habit. It doesn't actually mean that you need to eat at that time.

Keep busy

When you are busy doing something, it makes fasting much easier compared to when sitting around and doing nothing. Many people prefer to do a 24 hour fast on days they know that they will be busy.

Here is a research study that will open your eyes to the feelings of hunger: To make this easy to understand, my notes are at the beginning and are shaded.

Study: Effect of calorie restriction on subjective ratings of appetite.[1]

People in the Healthy diet (control) group who did not lose any weight had the same levels of hunger as the people in the other three groups that lost weight. This is another example where you realize how much of hunger is mental.

---

[1]Pennington Biomedical Research Center, Baton Rouge, LA, USA. J Hum Nutr Diet. 2009 Apr;22(2):141-7.

Background: Energy or calorie restriction (CR) has consistently been shown to produce weight loss and have beneficial health effects in numerous species, including primates and humans. Most individuals, however, are unable to sustain weight losses induced through reductions in energy intake, potentially due to increased hunger levels. The effects that prolonged CR has on subjective aspects of appetite have not been well studied. Thus, the present study tested the effect of 6 months of caloric restriction on appetite in healthy, overweight men and women.

Methods: Forty-eight overweight men and women with a body mass index between 25-29.9 took part in a 6-month study and were randomized into one of four groups:

- Healthy diet (control)

- 25% Calorie Restriction (CR)

- 12.5% Calorie Restriction plus exercise (12.5% increased energy expenditure; CR + EX)

- Low-calorie diet [LCD; (890 kcal day) until 15% of initial body weight was lost, then maintenance].

Appetite markers (i.e. hunger, fullness, desire to eat, etc.) were assessed weekly during a fasting state.

Results: Body weight was significantly reduced in all three energy-restricted groups (CR; CR + EX; and LCD), indicating that participants were adherent to their energy restriction regimen, whereas the healthy diet control group remained weight stable.

Despite these significant weight losses, appetite ratings of participants in the three energy-restricted groups at month 6 were similar to the weight stable control group.

Conclusions: Calorie Restriction regimens with low fat diets producing significant weight losses have similar effects on appetite markers over a 6-month time period compared to a weight stable control group.

20   Teenagers And A Dog Trainer

Skipping Meals is easy. Trying to figure out diet books and unique diets is complicated

Short answer: Teenagers should be treated as adults. I really believe this.

I think this book should be required reading in High School Health class. A book that helps people answer a problem that will most likely affect them their entire life is too valuable to let them find by chance.

I understand that geometry should be taught as a class, but I never use it and neither will the vast majority of students. On the other hand, everyone needs to understand what is in this book. Think what a gift it would have been if you learned at age 16, the easy medical facts about how to stay thin.

The obesity problem has spread to teenagers just like adults. How valuable would it be to have every teenager in the country read this book? This could save the country a whopping amount of money in future healthcare costs by reducing obesity.

Are parents sending the wrong message?

Yes, parents usually are sending the wrong message.

Here is a conversation I had a couple weeks ago. I included it because I have conversations like this all the time.

I was talking with a woman about her 2 daughters. One daughter is thin and one daughter is not.

She told me about how she took the overweight daughter to a dietician/nutritionist and with the advice given; the overweight daughter is eating 3 meals and 2 snacks per day.

I asked her why she is going to feed the overweight daughter more if she wants her to lose weight? She looked at me rather puzzled, but I could tell that she was thinking about what I had just said.

Then I asked her to tell me about the thin daughter. She said that the thin daughter usually doesn't eat breakfast and frequently leaves the house without eating. When she was telling me this, she was saying it as if there was a problem. She also said that she is always trying to get the thin daughter to eat.

So my next question was this, I asked if the thin daughter was too skinny or if she looked good. She said that the thin daughter looked great.

If she looks great, I asked why then are you trying to make her eat when she is not hungry? Do you no longer want her to look great?

Now I really had her thinking. It was like I could see the wheels turning in her head as she mulled over what I was asking.

Then I went back to my questioning, and why are you feeding your overweight daughter more times per day?

By this time she was really starting to understand the errors of her ways. So I continued and said this.

I don't know about you, but if I were an overweight girl in high school, I would not want to be carrying snacks in my backpack because I was told I have to eat every few hours to lose weight. This will focus the girl's whole life on food.

I would suggest the overweight daughter eat less, just like the thin daughter. I would have her skip some meals and tell her to enjoy what she eats when she does eat. If she is in a hurry and on her way out of the house to hang out with friends, or go to school or whatever, don't tell her she needs to eat first, because she really doesn't.

It was like a light bulb went off in her head. She suddenly got it. Now, imagine how much more this will sink in and be of value when the overweight daughter reads this book.

Eating Disorders

Won't fasting and skipping meals cause eating disorders? NO

I haven't seen that happen. There is always going to be a percentage of the population that has eating disorders. I just don't think fasting causes them.

Learning to get in tune with your body and not stuffing yourself full of food just because it is a certain time of the day is invaluable information. Learning how to control one's weight prevents all kinds of health problems.

Reading the information in this book helps teenagers learn to avoid the number one health risk in non-poverty countries, which is obesity. By the way, now some very poor countries are also developing obesity.

There are going to be people who have eating disorders no matter what is recommended to them. I was watching the History Channel around Christmas one year and a show was talking about nuns in the 1400's who were anorexic and another nun that had bulimia. Eating disorders commonly co-exist with other psychological disorders as well.

I can tell you this, anorexia and bulimia are serious disorders that medical professionals are equipped to treat. I have concern for these people and would refer them to the proper professionals if I encountered them. That being said, however, there are way more people who are suffering from obesity than both these conditions combined and this book is about helping people get the answers to fix their problems that deal with being overweight, how to get lean and how to stay lean.

Dog Trainer Mike Dizak

You are probably wondering why the heck I am talking about a dog trainer. Keep reading, it will become glaringly obvious.

I have a patient/friend, Mike Dizak, who is a professional fighter and dog trainer. He normally trains personal protection dogs, but had gotten a small dog from someone. He gave us this dog (Chihuahua) that we had for about 6 weeks before we gave it to some family friends.

Mike was training for a fight in Costa Rica and I hadn't seen him for a while. He came over to say hi after we had the dog for about a month. Right away, he noticed the dog had gained weight.

Mike picked up the dog and looked at its stomach. Mike said to look at how the stomach is hanging lower and then he pointed to the dogs lower ribs by the hind legs. *Mike compared the dog to a human, if you can't see those lower ribs; there is too much body fat.*

Mike said that this is how he feeds his dogs. If he can't see those lower ribs, he cuts back on how much he feeds the dogs and cuts back to 1 feeding per day. Normally he does 2 feedings per day. Don't let the dog free feed all day long he added.

Notice that Mike's advice was very simple. Feed the dog less. Cut from 2 feedings per day to 1 feeding per day.

Now notice what Mike did not say.

Mike did NOT say "Feed the dog 3 meals and 3 snacks per day to lean the dog up?" Mike didn't say this either, "Drop the dog's carb intake?" and Mike certainly did NOT say this "Reduce the dog's fat intake?"

The dog trainer's method was simple and that is what he does with his dogs because it works. Cut back on the feedings. Simple and effective.

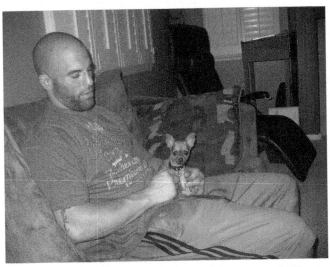

Mike Dizak professional fighter and dog trainer, 2010

21 Ramadan And Greek Fasting

Fasting saves you money and requires no payments or start-up fees

Ramadan is the religiously motivated fasts that people who follow the Islamic religion participate in. Ramadan is a 28 - 30 day fast in which food and drink are prohibited during the daylight hours (an average of 12 hours per day).

Greek Orthodox Christians fast for a total of 180 – 200 days each year, which include Lent (48 days before Easter), Assumption (15 days in August) and Nativity Fast (40 days before Christmas).

Both Ramadan and Greek Orthodox Christians experience benefits from the fasts including lowering of LDL (bad) cholesterol and lowering of body mass (when calorie intake is lowered).

Here are some studies that show the benefits of these two religious fasting periods: To make this easy to understand, my notes are at the beginning and are shaded.

Study: Effects of Greek Orthodox Christian Church fasting on serum lipids and obesity.[1]

Fasting lowered bad cholesterol (LDL) and total cholesterol.

---

[1]Department of Social Medicine, University of Crete, School of Medicine, P,O Box 1393, Iraklion 71110, Crete, Greece. BMC Public Health. 2003 May 16;3:16.

Methods: 120 Greek adults were followed longitudinally for one year. Sixty fasted regularly in all fasting periods (fasters) and 60 did not fast at all (controls). The three major fasting periods under study were: Christmas (40 days), Lent (48 days) and Assumption (August, 15 days). A total of 6 measurements were made during one year including pre- and end-fasting blood collection, serum lipoprotein analyses and anthropometric measurements.

Results: Statistically significant end-fasting total (-12.5%) and LDL cholesterol (-15.9%) differences were found in fasters. No change was found in control subjects.

Conclusions: Adherence to Greek Orthodox fasting periods contributes to a reduction in the blood lipid profile including a non-significant reduction in HDL cholesterol and possible impact on obesity.

Study: Effects of intermittent fasting on serum lipid levels, coagulation status and plasma homocysteine levels.[2]

Fasting improved cholesterol levels.

Background: During Ramadan, Muslims fast during the daylight hours for a month. The duration of restricted food and beverage intake is approximately 12 h/day which makes Ramadan a unique model of intermittent fasting.

---

[2]Department of Biochemistry, School of Medicine, Maltepe University, Istanbul, Turkey. Ann Nutr Metab. 2005 Mar-Apr;49(2):77-82. Epub 2005 Mar 29.

Conclusion: Our results demonstrate that intermittent fasting led to some beneficial changes in serum HDL and plasma homocysteine levels, and the coagulation status.

Study: Effects of Ramadan fasting on physical performance and metabolic, hormonal, and inflammatory parameters in middle-distance runners.[3]

Ramadan involves people getting less sleep than they normally would, which obviously causes sleepiness. Even though these people fasted during daylight hours, their testosterone/cortisol ratio stayed the same indicating that fasting did not harm testosterone levels.

The Ramadan fasting (RF) period is associated with changes in sleep habits.

In 8 middle-distance athletes (25.0 +/- 1.3 years), a maximal aerobic velocity (MAV) test was performed 5 days before Ramadan Fasting (day -5), and on days 7 and 21 of Ramadan Fasting.

The same days, saliva samples were collected to determine cortisol and testosterone concentrations before and after the Maximal Aerobic Velocity test.

Plasma levels of interleukin (IL)-6, a mediator of sleepiness and energy availability, were determined. We also evaluated changes in metabolic and hormonal parameters, mood state, and nutritional and sleep profiles. Testosterone/cortisol ratio values did not change significantly.

---

[3]Department of Physiology, IMASSA, Bretigny-sur-Orge, France. Appl Physiol Nutr Metab. 2009 Aug;34(4):587-94.

22   Hormones

Some people want to know about hormone levels, however, most people could care less, and just want to know how to lose weight. That is why the basics about what to do and how to do it are not located in the last chapter.

This chapter covers some of the main hormones that have to do with weight loss. You will quickly find that the fasting recommendations in Fat Loss the Truth improve the hormone levels that help you lose weight.

Insulin – (think fat storage)

If you want to burn body fat, lower your insulin levels.

Insulin, which is produced in the pancreas, helps tissue uptake blood sugar (glucose). Insulin also stimulates storage of triglycerides and protein. After a meal, insulin is released and the body goes into storage mode. This is called being in the Fed state.

(The Fasting state inhibits the release of insulin and allows the body to burn stored fat for fuel)

A high insulin level, accompanied by normal blood sugar, may indicate that the pancreas is working extra hard to keep the blood sugar level down. This condition is called insulin resistance and is very common with obese people and is usually corrected by losing weight and fasting.

So if insulin causes cells to uptake sugar from the blood, what effect does insulin have on body fat? Insulin stops the use of fat as an energy source. It does this by inhibiting the release of another hormone called glucagon.

The body burns fat for energy when insulin is absent. Here is research that says fasting lowers insulin levels: To make this easy to understand, my notes are at the beginning and are shaded.

Study: Effect of intermittent fasting and refeeding on insulin action in healthy men.[1]

Insulin function is improved by fasting times of only 20 hours. To lose body fat it is important for insulin to function correctly and not be resistant. When insulin is resistant it is at a high level in the blood, which prevents fat burning. The great news is that fasting lowers insulin, which allows fat burning to take place.

Insulin resistance is currently a major health problem. This may be because of a marked decrease in daily physical activity during recent decades combined with constant food abundance.

This lifestyle collides with our genome, which was most likely selected in the late Paleolithic era (50,000-10,000 BC) by criteria that favored survival in an environment characterized by fluctuations between periods of feast and famine. The theory of thrifty genes states that these fluctuations are required for optimal metabolic function.

We mimicked the fluctuations in eight healthy young men; by subjecting them to intermittent fasting every second day for 20 hours for 15 days.

---

[1]Dept. of Muscle Research Centre, The Panum Institute, University of Copenhagen, Denmark. J Appl Physiol. 2005 Dec;99(6):2128-36. Epub 2005 Jul 28.

This experiment is the first in humans to show that intermittent fasting increases insulin-mediated glucose uptake rates, and the findings are compatible with the thrifty gene concept.

From what I have seen and the research I have read, fasting is the fastest way to lower insulin levels, which leads to the burning of fat.

Remember from the "Different Ways to Fast" chapter that our sweet spot with fasting is 18 to 24 hours and 70% of the Reduction in Insulin Levels occurs in the first 24 hours of fasting.

Here is a little more information about insulin resistance.

When everything is working correctly, a small amount of insulin is used to do its job. When this small amount of insulin can no longer get the job done, more insulin is released. This is called insulin resistance and is highly connected to weight gain. Realize that abdominal fat is more resistant to insulin than any other fat in the body. This gives more meaning to Jack LaLanne's statement that your waistline is your lifeline.

Many health issues besides weight gain are also connected to this insulin problems such as: diabetes, high blood pressure, atherosclerosis, fatigue, high cholesterol, fatty liver disease, high triglycerides, candida and polycystic ovary disease. Other issues caused are an acidic pH and an increased amount of inflammation in the body.

When I look at blood work of people with insulin and sugar problems, I frequently see a need for magnesium and zinc and also see imbalances in the ratio of calcium and phosphorus. I also commonly see a drop in testosterone and DHEA as well.

Here is another study showing improved insulin levels: To make this easy to understand, my notes are at the beginning and are shaded.

Study: Improvements in body composition, glucose tolerance, and insulin action induced by increasing energy expenditure or decreasing energy intake.[2]

Calorie Restriction improved insulin levels and caused people to lose fat.

Increases in Exercise energy expenditure without compensatory changes in food intake and Calorie Restriction both decrease body weight and fat mass, which, in turn, improve glucoregulatory function.

Forty-eight sedentary 50- to 60-y-old men and women, most of whom were overweight, underwent 12 months of Exercise, Calorie Restriction, or a healthy lifestyle control period.

Body weight, total fat mass, and visceral fat volume decreased similarly in the Exercise and Calorie Restriction groups but did not change in the Healthy Lifestyle group.

Likewise, insulin sensitivity index and the oral glucose tolerance test glucose and insulin improved similarly in the Exercise and Calorie Restriction groups and remained unchanged in the Healthy Lifestyle group.

In conclusion, weight losses induced by exercise and by calorie restriction are effective means for improving glu-

[2]Division of Geriatrics and Nutritional Sciences, Department of Internal Medicine, Washington University School of Medicine, St. Louis, MO 63110, USA. J Nutr. 2007 Apr;137(4):1087-90.

cose tolerance and insulin action in nonobese, healthy, middle-aged men and women; however, it does not appear that exercise training-induced weight loss results in greater improvements than those that result from Calorie Restriction.

Glucagon – (think fat burning)

Glucagon is a hormone that raises blood sugar (glucose) levels by converting stored sugar into sugar that enters the blood. Glucagon also adjusts how fast sugar is being made by way of a process called lipolysis (the breakdown of fats which can be used for energy).

Glucagon has the opposite effect of insulin. Glucagon helps fat burning while insulin helps fat storage. You need both glucagon and insulin because they are part of a feedback system that keep blood sugar levels stable.

During the periods you are fasting, your muscles are burning fat for energy. The largest increase in plasma free fatty acids occurs in the first 24 hours with greatest release of fats happening between 18 and 24 hours.

Growth Hormone – (think lower body fat)

Growth Hormone, like testosterone, is a natural hormone that is produced in your body. These hormones usually make the headlines when an athlete takes them because both hormones are banned substances for athletes.

Growth hormone has many functions and many that are most likely unknown. For the purpose of this book, we will take into account that *growth hormone causes people to lose body fat by way of lipolysis. Lucky for us, fasting increases growth hormone levels naturally.*

As one ages, they produce less growth hormone. Just so you know, some doctors are prescribing growth hormone to older people to increase vitality and make them feel younger. This treatment is very expensive and there are potential side effects, plus a lot is still unknown about the long-term results of this treatment. Some doctors swear by it and others are highly opposed to it at this point in time.

The good thing is that you can naturally increase your level of growth hormone levels with out the potential side effects of the treatments. *Growth Hormone is increased through fasting, which causes you to lose body fat.*

There is a bunch of research that shows fasting improving Growth Hormone levels. To make these studies easy to understand, my notes are at the beginning and are shaded.

Study: Augmented growth hormone (GH) secretory burst frequency and amplitude mediate enhanced GH secretion during a two-day fast in normal men.[3]

Growth Hormone levels rose 5-fold with fasting!

Serum Growth Hormone concentrations are increased in fasted human subjects. We investigated the dynamic mechanisms underlying this phenomenon in nine normal men by analyzing serum Growth Hormone concentrations measured in blood obtained at 5-min intervals over 24 hours on a control (fed) day and on the second day of a fast.

---

[3]Department of Medicine, University of Virginia, Charlottesville 22908. J Clin Endocrinol Metab. 1992 Apr;74(4):757-65.

Two days of *fasting induced a 5-fold increase in the 24-hour endogenous Growth Hormone production rate.*

This enhanced Growth Hormone production rate was accounted for *by 2-fold increases in the number of Growth Hormone secretory bursts per 24 hours and the mass of Growth Hormone secreted per burst* (maximal rates of Growth Hormone release attained within a burst).

Growth Hormone was secreted in complex volleys composed of multiple discrete secretory bursts. These secretory volleys were separated by shorter intervals of secretory quiescence in the fasted than fed state.

Similarly, within volleys of GH release, constituent individual *secretory bursts occurred more frequently during the fast* [every 33 +/- 0.64 (fasted) vs. every 44 +/- 2.0 min (fed)].

Study: Impact of fasting on growth hormone signaling and action in muscle and fat.[4]

Fasting causes the breakdown of fats that can be used for energy. People that get prescription growth hormone do not get the full fat loss benefits unless they also use fasting. Fasting is the key that unlocks the fat burning gates and is free and easy to use.

Context: Whether GH promotes IGF-I production or lipolysis depends on nutritional status, but the underlying mechanisms remain unknown.

[4]Medical Department M, Aarhus Sygehus, Norrebrogade 44, DK-8000 Aarhus, Denmark. J Clin Endocrinol Metab. 2009 Mar;94(3):965-72. Epub 2008 Dec 9.

Objective: To investigate the impact of fasting on GH-mediated changes in substrate metabolism, insulin sensitivity, and signaling pathways.

Subjects: Ten healthy men participated.

Intervention: A Growth Hormone pharmaceutical preparation administered 1. after absorption, 2. in the fasting state (37.5 hours).

Main Outcome Measures: Metabolic clearance rate (MCR) of Growth Hormone, substrate metabolism, and insulin sensitivity were measured.

Results: *Fasting was associated* with reduced MCR of GH *(increased growth hormone levels)*, and enhanced lipolysis.

Conclusion: The combination of fasting and GH exposure translates into enhanced lipolysis, reduced IGF-I activity and insulin sensitivity.

Study: The protein-retaining effects of growth hormone during fasting involve inhibition of muscle-protein breakdown.[5]

Fasting increases growth hormone levels which helps keep muscle tissue intact.

The metabolic response to fasting involves a series of hormonal and metabolic adaptations leading to protein conservation. An increase in the serum level of growth hormone (GH) during fasting has been well substantiated. The present study was designed to test the hypothesis that GH

---

[5]Medical Department M, Aarhus Kommunehospital, Denmark. Diabetes. 2001 Jan;50(1):96-104.

may be a principal mediator of protein conservation during fasting and to assess the underlying mechanisms.

Eight normal subjects were examined on four occasions:

1. in the basal postabsorptive state (basal),

2. after 40 hours of fasting (fast),

3. after 40 hours of fasting with somatostatin suppression of GH (fast-GH), and

4. after 40 hours of fasting with suppression of GH and exogenous GH replacement (fast+GH).

In summary, we find that suppression of GH during fasting leads to a 50% increase in urea-nitrogen excretion, together with an increased net release and appearance rate of phenylalanine across the forearm.

Study: Effects of GH on protein metabolism during dietary restriction in man.[6]

This is another study that points out that fasting increases Growth Hormone levels which helps keep muscle tissue intact.

An increase in the serum level of growth hormone (GH) during fasting has been well substantiated.

---

[6]Medical Department M (Endocrinology and Diabetes), Aarhus Kommunehospital, Aarhus, Denmark. Growth Horm IGF Res. 2002 Aug;12(4):198-207.

Growth Hormone has potent protein anabolic actions, as evidenced by a significant decrease in lean body mass and muscle mass in chronic GH deficiency.

The present review outlines current knowledge about the role of GH in the metabolic response to fasting, with particular reference to the effects on protein metabolism.

Bursts of Growth Hormone secretion seem to be of seminal importance for the regulation of protein conservation during fasting.

Apart from the possible direct effects of GH on protein dynamics, a number of additional anabolic agents, such as insulin, insulin-like growth factor-I, and free fatty acids (FFAs), are activated. Taken together the effects of GH on protein metabolism seem to include both stimulation of protein synthesis and inhibition of breakdown.

Study: Obesity attenuates the Growth Hormone response to exercise.[7]

This shows that thin people produce more growth hormone than fat people. Since Growth Hormone helps you lose body fat, the more fat that a person loses, the more growth hormone they will produce.

Resting serum Growth Hormone (GH) concentrations are decreased in obesity. In nonobese (NonOb) individuals, acute exercise of sufficient intensity increases GH levels; however, conflicting data exist concerning the GH response to exercise in obese individuals.

---

[7]Department of Exercise Science, Syracuse University, New York 13244, USA. J Clin Endocrinol Metab. 1999 Sep;84(9):3156-61.

To examine the exercise-induced GH response in obese individuals, we studied 8 NonOb, 11 lower body obese (LBO), and 12 upper body obese (UBO) women before, during, and after 30 min of treadmill exercise at 70% oxygen consumption peak.

Blood samples were taken every 5 min (0700-1300 hours) and were analyzed for GH concentrations. The impact of 16 weeks of aerobic exercise training on the GH response to exercise was also examined in the obese women.

In response to exercise, the 6-hour integrated GH concentration was significantly greater in the NonOb women than in either of the obese groups. No differences were found between the LBO and UBO women.

This increase was attributed to a greater mass of Growth Hormone secreted per pulse in the Non Obese women.

After 16 weeks of aerobic training, maximal oxygen consumption increased, but no significant change in body composition occurred in the 10 obese women who completed the training. No change was observed in the GH response to exercise after training.

In conclusion, the GH response to exercise was attenuated in the obese women compared to NonOb women. Short term aerobic training improved fitness, but did not increase the GH response to exercise.

Study: Massive weight loss restores 24-hour growth hormone release profiles and serum insulin-like growth factor-I levels in obese subjects.[8]

After a massive weight loss in obese people, growth hormone and insulin levels returned to normal.

In the present study, we 1) determined whether the impaired spontaneous 24-hour Growth Hormone (GH) secretion as well as the blunted GH response to provocative testing in obese subjects are persistent disorders or transient defects reversed with weight loss and 2) investigated 24-hour urinary GH excretion and basal levels of insulin-like growth factor-I (IGF-I), IGF-binding protein-3 (IGFBP-3), as well as insulin in obese subjects before and after a massive weight loss.

We studied 18 obese subjects; 18 normal age-, and sex-matched control subjects; and 9 reduced weight obese subjects after a diet-induced average weight loss of 30.3 +/- 4.6 kg.

In obese subjects, 24-hour spontaneous GH secretion and serum IGF-I levels were inversely related to abdominal fat and percent body fat, respectively.

The decreased 24-hour spontaneous GH release profiles, the decreased GH responses to insulin-induced hypoglycemia and L-arginine, the decreased basal IGF-I levels and IGF-I/IGFBP-3 molar ratio, as well as the elevated in-

[8]Department of Internal Medicine and Endocrinology, Hvidovre University Hospital, Denmark.   J Clin Endocrinol Metab.   1995 Apr;80(4):1407-15.

sulin levels were returned to normal after a massive weight loss in the obese subjects.

In conclusion, the present study has shown reversible defects in 24-hour spontaneous GH release profiles, basal IGF-I levels, and the IGF-I/IGFBP-3 molar ratio in obese subjects. The recovery of the 24-hour GH release points to an acquired transient defect rather than a persistent preexisting disorder.

23   Blood Sugar

Diabetics - Don't use Fasting unless you work with your doctor. Type 1 diabetics may not be able to use fasting. I don't have much experience with this but have heard accounts of success from some. Type 2 diabetics may get good benefits from fasting. Remember to check with your doctor and proceed at a slow pace while closely monitoring your blood sugar.

Hypoglycemia - Is when your blood sugar level drops. It does exist, however it is very uncommon.

Typically, what happens is people have in their mind that they must eat frequently or they get low blood sugar. They have developed a learned response and convinced themselves that they have to eat every 3 hours or they have a problem. This is rarely more than your mind playing tricks on you.

Here is how the scene usually plays out. I have a patient that says they can't fast because they have hypoglycemia. I explain that I used to think the same thing about myself until I got a glucometer and tested my blood sugar. What I found was that my blood sugar really wasn't going low. Once I saw the actual measurement of my blood sugar, I realized it was my mind playing tricks on me and I never have felt hypoglycemic symptoms again.

Then I explain that hypoglycemia exists, but is not common. Normal people can fast for 1 day easily without having low blood sugar. I then suggest that they start with a simple 14 - hour fast or buy their own glucometer and start testing their blood sugar.

So then what happens is usually one of these two things.

In both cases they realize they were mentally creating the symptoms. 1. They start fasting and they feel fine. 2. They get a glucometer and see that their blood sugar is not going low and then they realize the symptoms were all in their head.

The third thing that I have seen is they actually do have a blood sugar level that drops. In these cases, I would recommend supplements to start with that help with blood sugar. There are a number of supplements that I would potentially use.

I would also tell the patient to continue using a glucometer to see if there is improvement after they start the supplements. Lastly, don't do anything pertaining to long periods of time with fasting unless you resolve these blood sugar issues. Consult your doctor and they may be able to provide you with more advice.

As a side note, I have seen remarkable changes using supplementation to help give support for blood sugar issues. However, I feel a doctor should help assist the patient with these issues. Therefore, I am not going into great detail, but here is an example to wet your whistle and show you there is a basis for what I am saying. Finding a doctor with knowledge of supplements and blood sugar can also be a challenge but very beneficial when you find one.

Study: Effects of acute chromium supplementation on postprandial metabolism in healthy young men.[1]

My own suspicions about this study are that the people who didn't respond were probably not low in chromium in the first place. I do significant amounts of blood testing and I will say that minerals such as chromium, iodine, zinc and magnesium are very common to be low and can cause many problems in the body.

Chromium potentiates the action of insulin in the cell and improves glucose (sugar) tolerance.

Conclusion: *Chromium supplementation showed an effect on postprandial (after the meal) sugar metabolism in most people.*

---

[1]INW Nutrition Biology, Department of Agriculture and Food Sciences, Swiss Federal Institute of Technology Zurich, Switzerland. J Am Coll Nutr. 2004 Aug;23(4):351-7.

What about Hypoglycemia?

Study: Effect of fasting on young adults who have symptoms of hypoglycemia in the absence of frequent meals.[2]

Were the symptoms such as irritation and shakiness all mental? I think so, since the lowest blood sugar recorded was 66 and doctors typically state that symptoms from hypoglycemia do not start until the blood sugar drops below 55. The conclusion said that these people could go ahead and fast.

Background and Objectives: Among otherwise healthy adults, there is a subgroup of individuals who develop symptoms of hypoglycemia during episodes of food restriction. The aim of the present study was to investigate whether such individuals develop hypoglycemia or react abnormally in other metabolic aspects during a 24-hour fast.

Subjects and Methods: Ninety medical students were asked if they wanted to participate. Sixteen were selected; none dropped out. A 24-hour fast was performed at a hospital ward. Blood samples and questionnaires were taken at eight specific times.

Result: During the fast, the sensitive group reported significantly higher scores on 'irritation' and 'shakiness'. However, no hypoglycemia occurred and the lowest detected

[2]Department for Clinical Science, Intervention and Technology, Karolinska Institutet, Huddinge, Department of Pediatrics, Karolinska University Hospital, Stockholm, Sweden. Eur J Clin Nutr. 2008 Jun;62(6):721-6. Epub 2007 May 16.

blood glucose concentration was 3.7 mmol/l (66 mg/dl). There were no differences between the groups in plasma glucose, cortisol, growth hormone (GH), insulin, beta-hydroxy-butyrate (beta-OH) and lactate levels. The blood pressures and heart rates were also similar.

Conclusions: *Adults, despite subjective signs of hypoglycemia, can fast without any metabolic or endocrine derangement.*

High Blood Sugar ages you at a much faster rate. This is something I witnessed in my practice. South Carolina had the highest diabetes rates in the country so in turn I had a lot of patients with diabetes. I watched people that did not control their blood sugar age quickly.

Study: Evidence for the glycation hypothesis of aging from the food-restricted rodent model.[3]

Skipping meals causes calorie restriction, which slows the aging process.

Sugar has been proposed as a mediator of aging processes by means of glycation reactions resulting in advanced glycosylation end-products, thereby altering protein and DNA function.

Testing this provocative concept has a high priority in gerontologic research. In this study, food restriction of rats–a procedure which markedly retards aging processes–was used to test the glycation hypothesis.

---

[3]Department of Physiology, University of Texas Health Science Center, San Antonio. J Gerontol. 1989 Jan;44(1):B20-2.

Food-restricted rats were found to have a sustained plasma glucose (sugar) concentration and percentage glycosylation of hemoglobin significantly lower than those of ad libitum fed rats. These findings are consistent with and provide support for the glycation hypothesis.

Here is the often-quoted study from 1999 that says you should eat multiple meals per day. The study was performed on 7 people and limited insulin and blood sugar measurements were performed. Since this time, more specific research has been performed that take significantly more insulin and blood sugar measurements which give a better picture of what really is going on within the body. The other research shows that multiple meals raise blood sugar rather than lower it as shown in this study.

What follows is important to understand. The latest research shows that less meals is better than more meals:

Study: Acute appetite reduction associated with an increased frequency of eating in obese males.[4]

There are many things that were improved on in other studies as compared to the below study. For instance, this study only tested the blood every hour for 5 hours compared to another study which tested the blood every 15 minutes for 12 hours.

---

[4]Department of Physiology, University of Witwatersrand Medical School, Johannesburg, South Africa. Int J Obes Relat Metab Disord. 1999 Nov;23(11):1151-9.

With the additional testing, it was shown that eating multiple meals per day cause significantly higher blood sugar levels.

Objective: To investigate the effects of altered feeding frequencies on the relationship between perceived hunger and subsequent food intake and appetite control in obese men.

Design: Obese men reported in a fasted state in the morning to the laboratory where an isoenergetic pre-load comprising 70% carbohydrate, 15% protein, and 15% fat was given. This was administered either as a SINGLE meal, or divided evenly over 5 meals given hourly as a MULTI feeding pattern. Five hours after the first pre-load, an ad libitum test meal was given to determine whether there was a difference in the amount of energy that was consumed between the two eating patterns.

Subjects: Seven non-diabetic, non-smoking, unrestrained obese men were recruited for this study.

Results: When given a SINGLE pre-load, 27% more energy was consumed in the ad libitum test meal compared to that eaten after the MULTI pre-load.

This increase in food intake occurred despite no significant change in subjective hunger ratings.

Over the 315 min pre-load period, peak insulin concentrations were significantly higher on the SINGLE treatment than on the MULTI treatment.

Serum insulin remained elevated for longer on the MULTI meal treatment, resulting in no difference in the area under the insulin curves between the two feeding treatments.

My notes: Eating a single meal had a greater insulin spike, however the Multi meal plan kept insulin spiked for a longer period of time, which is much worse.

Conclusion: Obese males fed an isoenergetic pre-load subdivided into a multi-meal plan consumed 27% less at a subsequent ad libitum test meal than did the same men when given the pre-load as a single meal. Prolonged but attenuated increases in serum insulin concentration on the multi-meal program may facilitate this acute reduction in appetite.

What has occurred since this study?

More advanced studies have been done that show multiple meals cause higher overall blood sugar values. This is a bad thing if you are working on losing body fat.

What about a sense of fullness after eating?

Multiple meals are shown to be counterproductive.

Here is a more advanced and newer study:

Study: Effect of meal frequency on glucose and insulin excursions over the course of a day[5]

While eating the same amount of carbs, people that ate 6 meals per day had approximately 30% higher blood sugar values compared to eating 3 meals per day.

Let me say that again. Eating 6 meals per day was BAD. Six meals per day produced much Higher blood sugar val-

[5]The European e-Journal of Clinical Nutrition and Metabolism. Received 7 July 2010; accepted 5 October 2010. published online 25 October 2010.

ues compared to 3 meals per day. Not only is higher blood sugar bad for fat loss, it is also bad for your health and can potentially lead to type 2 diabetes.

Background & Aims: This study characterized the glucose and insulin responses to temporal alterations in meal frequency, and alterations in the macronutrient composition.

Methods: Eight subjects underwent three separate 12-hour meal tests: three high carbohydrate (3CHO) meals, 6 high carbohydrate meals (6CHO), 6 high-protein meals (6HP). Blood samples were taken at 15-min intervals. Integrated area under the curve concentrations for glucose and plasma insulin were determined for each meal condition.

Results: Peak glucose levels were highest on the 3CHO day; *however the 12 hour glucose AUC was higher eating 6 meals per day than 3 meals*, with no difference in the insulin response. The 6HP condition resulted in a decreased glucose and insulin compared to 6CHO.

Conclusions: In non-obese individuals, glucose levels remained elevated throughout the day with frequent CHO meals compared to 3CHO meals, without any differences in the insulin levels. Increasing the protein content of frequent meals attenuated both the glucose and insulin response. These findings of elevated glucose levels throughout the day warrant further research, particularly in overweight and obese individuals with and without type 2 diabetes.

24 Tips

1. YOU SHOULD LIFT WEIGHTS while doing a low calorie diet like fasting. This keeps your muscle tissue intact which keeps your metabolic rate high.

2. If I fast 18 to 24 hours, it is spread out over 2 days rather than going one day without eating.

3. I have noticed that eating a bunch of sugar right before starting the fast can promote hunger. Eating sugar in general for that matter, promotes hunger.

4. If you find yourself hungry during the fast, remember it is most likely mental and your mind playing tricks on you.

5. You will find that eating higher protein meals may help you diminish hunger.

6. Drink water. Many times people confuse thirst for hunger. Dehydration can mimic hunger.

7. Start meals with a salad. This is a great way to get in vegetables. This worked great for me in college. I got in veggies and found that I naturally stopped eating deserts because I wasn't hungry for them. When I did have a desert, which wasn't common, it was usually something I really enjoyed and just 1 serving.

8. Don't snack. I feel that eating small snacks throughout the day just makes me hungry and the research I posted in this book shows the same thing.

9. Sleep – getting 8 hours of sleep per night helps you get lean. Sleep is important and improves your hormone levels. Sleep is very important, don't overlook this point!

10. You don't have to conquer the world in one day. You can start at a slower pace if you really want to. For the first few days, cut out the snacks and just eat three meals. Then you can progress to the instructions in the "Different Ways to Fast" chapter.

25 Stuff Learned From Julie

There were many things that I tried to tell Julie she was wrong about, that I will now give her credit for being correct, before she can say "I told you so". I will also say that I am proud of her for going back to college and becoming a registered nurse at age 40.

1. Sun

Julie always said that she felt better overall after she sun tanned. I would say that the sun causes all these problems, yada, yada, yada.

Well, come to find out she was right and I was completely wrong.☺

With the vitamin D research that has come out in recent years, the majority of people are grossly vitamin D deficient. People get vitamin D primarily from the sun. Vitamin D deficiency is related to winter depression and a host of many other diseases. So getting vitamin D from being in the sun does make you feel better.

2. If you are not hungry, don't eat

There are so many times that I said it's time to eat and Julie said I am not hungry. So she would just not eat that meal. She didn't plan anything, rather just didn't eat if she wasn't hungry.

3. Eat what you want

Don't deprive yourself of anything, or you will just focus on it until you get it. Julie always ate what she wanted and didn't deprive herself. Her key was that she is a person that could naturally not overeat or just be satisfied with a little bit of something.

Many people who eat what they want can lose weight and stay thin by just incorporating the easy strategy of skipping meals.

4. Do what makes you happy

If you hate your job, do something else. This is a simple statement with deep meaning. If you don't like what you are doing, find something you like doing and do it.

I have worked 12-hour days for months at a time and made a lot of money and then had it all stolen from me by crooks and the government. Well I guess they are one in the same. ☺

The harder I worked, the more money I made; the less free time I had; and the more everyone else felt that my money I made from hard work belonged to them.

So I realize now, it's just like the Linkin Park song " In the end, it doesn't even matter". You can't take it with you. Why bust your tail knowing the government is just going to steal it from you anyway. Do what you enjoy while you are here. Chill out and have fun. Don't put all your time into work. Help as many people as you can that need help.

5. You should only wear clothes that make you feel great

You feel better about yourself when you like what you are wearing. This causes you to react better with other people.

6. Drive a vehicle that you like

We got a minivan to drive across the country. It had a lot of room and that is what we needed considering we had a 5 year old, a 6 week old and 2 cats. However, Julie hated it. She said that it didn't make her feel good about herself when we drove it. We sold it and got something else and she was happy about it.

It is just another example of doing things that make you feel good.

There is a lot to be said about putting yourself in a position where you are self confident and happy. I know people will say that you have to save for this or that and that happiness comes from within and I could go on and on.

Now really think about what I am saying.

Take a minute and remember how great you feel when you put on a certain special outfit you have. Everyone has some clothes that make him or her feel great. So why wouldn't you only wear clothes that make you feel great?????????

You will feel better about yourself and more self-confident. This is how you should live life. If it doesn't make you feel great, get rid of it.

7. Live for today

This one, Julie and I learned together.

I think of my grandpa. He was in World War II, came home, had 3 kids and worked for the electric company. He scrimped and saved. For instance, my father would tell me stories about their family eating the cheapest meat that his parents could buy so they could save money. He said it was like eating a piece of leather surrounded by a bunch of fat. They didn't spend a penny on any "luxuries" for themselves.

Then my grandpa got cancer, and died in his 50's. He saved his whole life for retirement. It was always about how great retirement will be. Then he never made it to retirement.

I can understand a savings plan for retirement up to a point. However, putting all your money into savings rather than enjoying your life is a different situation.

I can't even begin to tell you how many people I know who were screwed over by investing in the stock market with money they thought they would have for retirement. First came the tech market crash, then Enron, then the recession during the 2000's, and then finding out that the market was set up for bankers at the exclusion of us regular people. These people who worked hard for their money and spent years saving not only lost their retirement money, they never got to enjoy the money that they earned.

Live for today, do what makes you happy, wear clothes that make you feel great and drive a vehicle that you like.

8. Certain people, it is better to avoid

If someone has bad energy, avoid them. Don't argue with them, just smile and refrain from further contact with them.

There are people who will drag you down if you let them

and others who will draw you into arguments and their troubles. Avoid them. People who look to suck out all your energy. Avoid them.

One of the best things you can do is be positive for yourself and your family and friends. Realize, there are people who can turn you negative and make your life miserable. Avoid them.

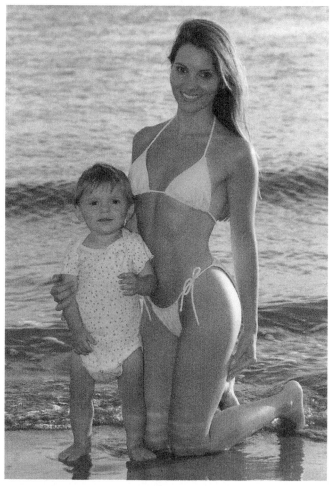

Julie Fitzgerald, age 30, with our first son, Colton.

26   Sleep

Sleep is very important to any weight loss and weight maintenance plan. People that get 8 hours of sleep lose more weight than those who don't.

Study: Insufficient sleep undermines dietary efforts to reduce adiposity.[1]

Sleeping for 8.5 hours per night resulted in 55% more weight loss than 5.5 hours per night.

Background: Sleep loss can modify energy intake and expenditure.

Objective: To determine whether sleep restriction attenuates the effect of a reduced-calorie diet on excess adiposity.

Patients: 10 overweight nonsmoking adults (3 women and 7 men) with a mean age of 41 years (SD, 5) and a mean body mass index of 27.4 kg/m² (SD, 2.0).

INTERVENTION: 14 days of moderate caloric restriction with 8.5 or 5.5 hours of nighttime sleep opportunity.

Measurements: The primary measure was loss of fat and fat-free body mass. Secondary measures were changes in substrate utilization, energy expenditure, hunger, and 24-hour metabolic hormone concentrations.

Results: Sleep curtailment decreased the proportion of weight lost as fat by 55% (1.4 vs. 0.6 kg with 8.5 vs. 5.5 hours

---

[1]The University of Chicago, Illinois, USA. Ann Intern Med. 2010 Oct 5;153(7):435-41.

of sleep opportunity, respectively) and increased the loss of fat-free body mass by 60% (1.5 vs. 2.4 kg). This was accompanied by markers of enhanced neuroendocrine adaptation to caloric restriction, increased hunger, and a shift in relative substrate utilization toward oxidation of less fat.

Conclusion: The amount of human sleep contributes to the maintenance of fat-free body mass at times of decreased energy intake. Lack of sufficient sleep may compromise the efficacy of typical dietary interventions for weight loss and related metabolic risk reduction.

27   Food Tastes Better

Fasting builds your self control

It has become so common nowadays for people to eat and snack all day and into the night. I fell under this ridiculous habit for several years.

One thing that I noticed is that food started to taste blah. There wasn't a lot of food that I thought really tasted good and more frequently than not, after a meal I would say, "I can't believe I ate that and didn't even like it."

Once you have started skipping meals, food will taste much, much better. It is like your tongue gets re-sensitized. Your meals will become much more enjoyable.

When you are truly hungry, (not just at your programmed time to eat) your food will taste much better.

You will find that you enjoy every bite after your fast and the funny thing is that many people also end up eating less when they sit down for a meal than they did before they started fasting.

Think of it this way. You have sex twice per day or twice per week. What feels better? If your older than 22, you probably chose twice per week. ☺

By the way, I was attending the annual American Anti-Aging Symposium for doctors in Las Vegas recently and one of the researchers presented information that says having sex every 48 hours is highly beneficial for your hormones. So I will pass along those recommendations on that time period for you. You know me, always looking out for your health. ☺

28   Exercise

You can't out exercise your mouth

Short Answer: Lift weights, stand up during the day rather than sitting. When you can walk, do so.

You should do resistive exercise, which can include lifting weights and/or bodyweight exercises such as pushups, pull-ups and squats.

I walked in the gym one day to see a fellow doctor acquaintance. He was a nice guy, short and slightly pudgy. I said that every time I come to the gym I see you. He said, wow, you don't come here very much because I don't see you that much.

His conversation turned to Burger King. He felt it was very important for me to know that BK was running some sort of special. I can't tell you what it was because this was several years ago, but he was very excited about it. He said he is working out so he can leave the gym and go to BK. I said that I am much too lazy for that and I would rather just change how I eat to stay lean.

What's funny about this was that I was lean and ripped with a 6 pack. He was far from lean. He was in the gym all the time and I rarely was. It was another realization that what you eat is WAY more important than how much time you spend exercising.

Make the most of your exercise time by lifting weights and realize that your calorie intake has way more to do with you becoming and staying lean than exercise. However, I will tell you this, you will benefit from lifting weights or doing bodyweight exercises such as pushups, pull-ups and squats when you utilize fasting. This keeps your muscles intact which keeps your metabolism high.

Stand Up

If possible, move your workstation so that you can stand rather than sit. When you stand, you use your leg muscles and postural muscles that burn energy.

Standing burns approximately 20 to 50 more calories per hour than sitting (It depends on how big you are). So, if you stand for 8 hours rather than sit, that can add up to a lot of calories per day. It makes a difference when you add standing into your lifestyle, no matter how big you are.

I have personally witnessed this with many patients and myself. Standing does make a difference.

My wife, Julie, ran the front desk in my office. When we first rented the office, it already had a tall desk where patients checked in. The desk was located where there was room for one chair. However, the chair was always in the way, so I moved it and she would stand during most of the time in the office. After a few months without the chair, she noticed that her butt was more toned from the standing.

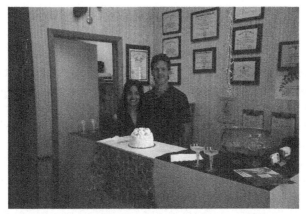

Julie Fitzgerald and Dr. John Fitzgerald in their office in 1997.
(This is the desk Julie would stand behind while at work)

I now work at home. So I got a pedestal to stand at while doing work. This makes a big difference.

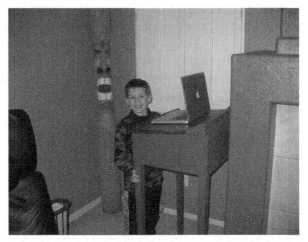

Logan Fitzgerald, age 7, standing at my pedestal/desk in our living room.

Walk when you can

You have a choice to move your body in your daily activities. For instance: I talk on the phone a lot. My consultations are done on the phone with people located all around the country and the world for that matter. So I use a cordless phone with a headset and walk laps (more like slowly strolling) inside my house and also around my back yard when I am on the phone. When I need to be in front of the computer, I stand. For me personally, this standing and walking made a big difference in my leanness. Plus I see a much better result doing this compared to when I was sitting all day and then doing some cardio on a treadmill later in the day. The standing and walking was more effective and it didn't take extra time to do, like the treadmill did.

If you are used to sitting all day as I once was, I remember being tired just switching to standing. So I started at a couple of hours per day standing, then kept increasing the time until I was doing it all day. I have many patients who have told me that they used to sit in front of the TV with their laptop computer on their lap and switched to standing with their computer on a pedestal while watching TV.

The numbers vary on how many calories one burns comparing sitting, standing and walking. There are variables such as how big the person is. Lets take some average numbers for a 150-pound person.

Sitting burns 80 calories per hour (There is plenty of research that says sitting contributes to obesity, diabetes, heart disease, certain cancers, and early death. These are added reasons to stand, beyond the purpose of this book, which is weight loss)

Standing burns 110 calories per hour

Walking burns 330 calories per hour

When all is said and done at the end of the day, standing and walking make a huge difference.

Here are several studies that talk about exercise. To make this easy to understand, my notes are at the beginning and are shaded.

Study: The daily walking distance of young doctors and their body mass index.[1]

A group of doctors who do the same job were followed around to measure their physical activity while at work. The thinner doctors walked four times farther than the other doctors each day.

Get up and move. Every little bit helps. When I park my car, I park far out away from everyone else and walk. The use it or lose it saying comes to mind.

Study: Metabolic responses to reduced daily steps in healthy nonexercising men.[2]

After 2 weeks of less walking, they became worse at metabolizing sugars and fats and developed decreased insulin

---

[1]Department of Medicine, Kantonsspital Baden, Switzerland. Eur J Intern Med. 2009 Oct;20(6):622-4. Epub 2009 Aug 6.

[2]Olsen RH, Krogh-Madsen R, Thomsen C, Booth FW, Pedersen BK. JAMA. 2008 Mar 19;299(11):1261-3.

sensitivity. Their body fat distribution changed and more fat was now located around their midsection.

Walking helps your body function better. People were tracked by how much they walk per day. Their steps were tracked with a pedometer. Normally, they walked an average of 10,501 steps per day and for 2 weeks cut back to an average of 1344 steps per day.

Study: Effect of exercise intensity on abdominal fat loss during calorie restriction in overweight and obese postmenopausal women: a randomized, controlled trial.[3]

With calorie restriction, total weight loss was similar whether or not the groups exercise, strengthening the point that the most important part about weight loss is calorie restriction. However, exercise helps you keep your muscle mass, which in the long run will help your metabolism.

Objective: This study showed whether aerobic exercise intensity affects the loss of abdominal fat and improvement in cardiovascular disease risk factors under conditions of equal energy deficit in women with abdominal obesity.

Design: This was a randomized trial in 112 overweight and obese postmenopausal women assigned to one of three 20-wk interventions of equal energy deficit:

[3]Section on Gerontology and Geriatric Medicine, J Paul Sticht Center on Aging, Department of Internal Medicine, Wake Forest University Health Sciences, Winston-Salem, NC 27157, USA. Am J Clin Nutr. 2009 Apr;89(4):1043-52. Epub 2009 Feb 11.

- Calorie restriction (CR only)

- CR plus moderate-intensity aerobic exercise (CR + moderate-intensity)

- CR plus vigorous-intensity exercise (CR + vigorous-intensity)

The diet was a controlled program of underfeeding during which meals were provided at individual calorie levels (approximately 400 kcal/d).

Exercise (3 d/wk) involved treadmill walking at an intensity of 45-50% (moderate-intensity) or 70-75% (vigorous-intensity) of heart rate reserve.

Results: *Average weight loss for the 95 women who completed the study was 12.1 kg and was not significantly different across groups.* Maximal oxygen uptake increased more in the CR + vigorous-intensity group than in either of the other groups. *The CR-only group lost relatively more lean mass than did either exercise group.* All groups showed similar decreases in abdominal visceral fat. However, changes in visceral fat were inversely related to increases in O(2)max. Changes in lipids, fasting glucose or insulin, and 2-hour glucose and insulin areas during the oral-glucose-tolerance test were similar across treatment groups.

Study: Successful long-term weight maintenance: a 2-year follow-up.[4]

The ability to keep lost weight off after dieting is related to the ability to keep your muscle tissue intact while losing the weight in the first place.

Lifting weights while losing weight helps you retain your muscle tissue, which helps you keep the weight off.

Objective: To find factors associated with successful weight maintenance (WM) in overweight and obese subjects after a very low-calorie diet (VLCD).

Results: After 2 years of WM, 13 subjects were successful (<10% BW regain), and 90 were unsuccessful (>10% BW regain). At baseline, these groups were significantly different in BMI, respectively; and fat mass. Successful subjects increased their dietary restraint significantly more during the whole study period. Furthermore, %BW regain was associated with the amount of percentage body fat lost during VLCD, which indicates that the more fat lost, the better the Weight Maintenance, suggesting a fat free mass-sparing effect.

Discussion: Characteristics such as the ability to increase dietary restraint and maintain this high level of restraint, fat free mass sparing, and a relatively high baseline BMI and fat mass were associated with successful long-term WM (<10% regain after 2 years).

---

[4]Department of Human Biology, Maastricht University, P.O. Box 616, NL-6200 MD Maastricht, The Netherlands. Obesity (Silver Spring). 2007 May;15(5):1258-66.

Study: Training in the fasted state improves glucose tolerance during fat-rich diet.[5]

Burning fat is more effective when training in the fasted state. For regular people, there is no need to eat before training. There is a trade off. Exercising while being in a fasted state can decrease performance if extended endurance is the goal. However, most people want to burn fat when they exercise and the best way to do that is to exercise while in the fasted state.

If your goal is to burn fat, realize that common sense comes into play here. Eating more does not cause you to lose fat, and eating before exercise does not cause you to burn fat. Isn't that obvious? To lose fat, stop eating so frequently and so much!

Exercise in the fasted state markedly stimulates energy provision via fat oxidation (burning of fat). Therefore, we investigated whether exercise training in the fasted state is more potent than exercise in the fed state to rescue whole-body glucose tolerance and insulin sensitivity during a period of hyper-caloric fat-rich diet.

Healthy male volunteers (18-25 y) received a hyper-caloric, fat-rich diet for 6 weeks.

- Some of the subjects performed endurance exercise training in the fasted state (Fasted group).

[5]Research Centre for Exercise and Health, Department of Biomedical Kinesiology, K.U. Leuven, Leuven, Belgium. J Physiol. 2010 Nov 1;588(Pt 21):4289-302.

- Others ingested carbohydrates before and during the training sessions (carb group).

- The control group did not train (control group).

Body weight increased in the control group and the carb group, but not in Fasted group. The Fasted group also improved whole-body glucose tolerance and the Matsuda insulin sensitivity index.

Another benefit of the fasted group was that muscle GLUT4 protein content was increased in Fasted group (+28%) compared with both carb and control groups.

This study for the first time shows that fasted training is more potent than fed training to facilitate adaptations in muscle and to improve whole-body glucose tolerance and insulin sensitivity during hyper-caloric fat-rich diet.

Study: Exercise Dosing to Retain Resistance Training Adaptations in Young and Older Adults.[6]

This study showed that one training session per week may be enough for both young and old athletes to retain past strength gains.

In "The Ripped Books" chapter, I cover Clarence Bass's exercise schedule, which is one weightlifting session and one intense cardio session per week.

---

[6]Departments of 1Physiology and Biophysics, 2Physical Therapy, and 3Surgery, University of Alabama at Birmingham, Birmingham, Alabama 35294; 4Geriatric Research, Education, and Clinical Center, Birmingham Veterans Affairs Medical Center, Birmingham, Alabama 35233. Med Sci Sports Exerc. 2010 Dec 1.

This was a study to test the efficacy of Resistance training (RT) maintenance plans on muscle mass, myofiber size and type distribution, and strength. We hypothesized the minimum dose required to maintain RT-induced adaptations would be greater in old (60-75 y) vs. young (20-35 y).

Methods: Seventy adults participated in a two-phase exercise trial that consisted of RT 3 days/week for 16 weeks (Phase I)

Followed by a 32 week period (Phase II) with random assignment to detraining or one of two maintenance prescriptions:

Reducing the dose to 1/3 (1 time per week of RT) or 1/9 of that during Phase I.

Conclusions: We conclude that older adults require a higher dose of weekly loading than young to maintain myofiber hypertrophy attained during a progressive RT program; yet gains in specific strength among older adults were well-preserved and remained at or above levels of untrained young.

29   Models And Strippers

This chapter isn't full of research and a bunch of studies that I quote to prove my point. Rather, it is based on years of observation that I will humorously share with you.

My language shifts in this chapter. I put this chapter in simplistic terms. If you are sensitive or get offended easily, don't read this chapter.

Otherwise, lighten up, put a smile on your face and realize it is all in good fun to make you laugh and help you get the results you want. ☺

I have had many models and strippers as patients and even had some work for me. I have spent much time counseling people in the fitness industry also. I have made some observations that I will share with you because not a lot of people have been around models and strippers like I have, yet many people, especially girls, want to know what models and strippers do to stay lean.

I am frequently asked the question about some girl who is skinny and she supposedly eats what ever she wants. "Why is she so lucky?"

Well for one, she probably isn't as "lucky" as you many think. She is just not cramming her pie-hole full of food every chance she gets.

These girls usually eat what they want when they do eat, which is usually with other people around in a social setting. Their meals are social and enjoyable.

When they are alone, these girls are fasting for the most part. That's their big secret. Now you know, there is NO magic involved.

Contrast that with the fat chick that eats next to nothing in public when people are watching, she may even say that she is on a diet to let everyone know. Then she goes home and eats huge volumes of food when she is by herself.

The fat chick will say to me "Look at what she's eating and she is skinny. Look at what I am eating and I am fat...etc, etc." I always say, I bet she doesn't eat again until tomorrow afternoon. When are you going to eat again?

This is a simple, simple concept that so many overweight people do not comprehend. Eat and enjoy yourself, then don't eat. I will tell you that the skinny girl probably went home and didn't eat again until the next day in the afternoon. The fat chick probably went home and ate until she went to bed, then got up and started snacking again.

How to be a Model

Shut your mouth and quit eating so freaking much to start with! ☺ No kidding, right? I hope that made you laugh.

Seriously though, *Follow the outline in the "Different Ways to Fast" chapter. You will probably end up doing the "Combination of Both".*

When you do eat, focus on "real" foods. To be healthy, the less food you eat the more you should choose foods that are highly nutrient dense like vegetables. Did that make sense? Let me reword it for clarity. It is important to eat the most nutritious foods when you cut your calories and want to look your absolute best. When your body is healthier, you look better!

Pretty simple right? A diet of sugar, junk food, sodas, alcohol and cigarettes makes you look old and wrinkly way before your time. If you want to look like you were rode hard and put away wet, just eat like that and get as little sleep as possible and you will be well on your way to looking like something the cat dragged in.

If your diet is based on vegetables, fruits, wild caught fish such as salmon and grass-fed beef, you will be healthier and look better. When you start doing this you will notice that your skin will clear up, you hair will be shinier, your nails will be nicer and the whites of your eyes will be whiter. You will glow!

As a matter, of fact, one of the most effective ways to get rid of acne is to eat these healthy foods and eliminate the junk.

You can get skinny eating junk food as I mentioned in the "Junk Food Diet" chapter, but if you want to look your best, you will choose the healthiest foods with the most nutrients in them.

Strippers

Ok, here is the punch line. Yes, many strippers do a bunch of cocaine and speed. Strippers are generally up all night and sleep all day. Many of them smoke like a chimney and are frequently self-destructive types.

However, they are typically rail thin because they do not sit around eating all day. If they start eating too much and get fat, they get transferred to some club in the low rent district where they don't make much money and then move on to a different career. I thought I should do a study on this by interviewing every stripper in Vegas, but there wasn't enough time before this book was published. ☺

Strippers and models both eat infrequently for the most part and that is what keeps them lean. They usually eat 1 to 2 meals per day. Models usually pick healthier foods for the most part.

Here's another point: I have NEVER seen a skinny chick driving and eating, or stop at a fast food restaurant and eat in their car because they haven't eaten for a few hours. They sit down and socially enjoy their food, almost always from what I have seen. They are never in a rush to eat. If they are in a rush, they don't eat. Then they eat when they are no longer in a rush.

30   Troubleshooting

The weight is not coming off:

1. You are still eating too many calories

2. Your thyroid is slow

1. You are still eating too many calories

Here is the thing; you can still consume too much "Healthy" food. There are many different definitions of "Healthy" food so if you are not losing fat you will need to count your calories until you do start losing fat.

This is an exercise for you to see how many calories you are actually consuming and to learn to make better choices. For instance, you will find that veggies do not add up to high amounts of calories while nuts contain a substantial amount of calories.

Counting calories for a few weeks or more can really teach you how much food you can consume to lose weight.

Let's say that a good starting point for a man to lose weight is 1800 calories per day and for a woman would be 1200 calories per day. Divide that amount between the two meals. A man would have two meals of 900 calories for each meal and a woman would have 600 calories for each meal. Then measure your amount of food each meal so you are eating the appropriate amount of calories.

If you are losing weight each week, you are on track. If you are not losing weight, simply lower the calories on each meal you eat. *Remember this, if you are not losing weight, it is almost always because you are eating too many calories.*

Another method is to eat one plate of food at each meal. Do not get seconds. Eat one plate only. If you are losing weight, you are on track. If you are not losing weight, switch to a smaller plate of food.

If this sounds ridiculously easy, it should, because it is. The easier you make the process, the better.

Another method is to go longer periods of time fasting. You may go 36 or 48 hours without eating rather than 24 hours, but it is easier to simply reduce the size of your meals.

2. Your Thyroid is Slow

Sometimes people do have a slow thyroid gland, which causes a slow metabolism.

There are things to do for this such as make sure you are getting the necessary nutrients for your thyroid. It is common for people to be low in iodine, selenium, zinc and magnesium, which are all necessary for thyroid function. It is also common to have an adrenal problem that contributes to the overall problem of slow metabolism.

(I am currently writing a second book that describes tests you can do at home to check yourself for these problems)

31   Hypnosis

Short answer: Hypnosis is a tool that can make everything you do easier and more effective. It is most beneficial when it is added to any weight loss and weight management plan.

Lucky for you, skipping meals does not require the same amount of willpower that is needed for strict diets. When you combine skipping meals and hypnosis, you are making the weight loss process even easier for yourself.

Hypnosis is a scientifically validated method for training your unconscious mind to eat right.

As of 2011, most clinical hypnotherapists that specialize in weight loss charge approximately $200 per session and therapy is done over 6 to 12 sessions.

A viable and inexpensive alternative is hypnosis CDs that you can listen to on a daily basis.

After listening and recommending many hypnosis CD's, fellow master hypnotist Jake Shannon and myself recorded a series of hypnosis sessions that include many things both of us were looking for in hypnosis CD's.

Neither one of us liked the long format on many hypnosis CD's because it takes too much of a time commitment on a daily basis. Jake and I both found that people are willing to listen to a 15 to 20 minute session when they lay down at night to go to bed. It becomes something that patients look forward to.

It is now known that certain frequencies have healing properties and potentially can repair DNA damage. We edited in these frequencies that are on the cutting edge of anti-aging medicine and research. The tunes that you hear in the background of these hypnosis CD's are not just music. They are specific frequencies to induce certain brain waves while initiating healing within your cells as an added benefit to the hypnosis benefits that are taking place.

www.Hypfit.net

Research studies support hypnosis being used as part of a weight loss strategy. To make this easy to understand, my notes are at the beginning and are shaded.

Study: Hypnotic enhancement of cognitive-behavioral weight loss treatments–another meta-reanalysis.[1]

When utilizing Hypnosis, people lost more than double the weight than without Hypnosis.

In a 3rd meta-analysis of the effect of adding hypnosis to cognitive-behavioral treatments for weight reduction, additional data were obtained from authors of 2 studies, and computational inaccuracies in both previous meta-analyses were corrected. Averaged across posttreatment

[1]Department of Psychology, University of Connecticut, Storrs 06269-1020, USA. J Consult Clin Psychol. 1996 Jun;64(3):517-9.

and follow-up assessment periods, the *mean weight loss was 6.00 lbs. without hypnosis and 11.83 lbs. with hypnosis.*

The mean effect size of this difference was 0.66 SD. *At the last assessment period, the mean weight loss was 6.03 lbs. without hypnosis and 14.88 lbs. with hypnosis.* The effect size for this difference was 0.98 SD. Correlational analyses indicated that the *benefits of hypnosis increased substantially over time.*

Study: Hypnosis as an adjunct to cognitive-behavioral psychotherapy for obesity: a meta-analytic reappraisal.[2]

It was determined that Hypnosis provided only a small enhancement to weight loss. I added this study to show that different people have come up with different interpretations when looking over studies.

Kirsch, Montgomery, and Sapirstein (1995) meta-analyzed 6 weight-loss studies comparing the efficacy of cognitive-behavior therapy (CBT) alone to CBT plus hypnotherapy and concluded that *"the addition of hypnosis substantially enhanced treatment outcome".*

After correcting several transcription and computational inaccuracies in the original meta-analysis, these 6 studies yield a smaller mean effect size. Moreover, if 1 questionable study is removed from the analysis, the effect sizes become more homogeneous and the mean is no longer statistically significant. It is concluded that the addition of

[2]Obesity Research Center St. Luke's-Roosevelt Hospital Center Columbia University College of Physicians and Surgeons, New York, New York 10025, USA. J Consult Clin Psychol. 1996 Jun;64(3):513-6.

hypnosis to CBT for weight loss results in, at most, a small enhancement of treatment outcome.

Study: Effectiveness of hypnosis as an adjunct to behavioral weight management.[3]

People who used Hypnosis were more likely to achieve their goals and had long-term success.

This study examined the effect of adding hypnosis to a behavioral weight-management program on short- and long-term weight change.

One hundred nine subjects, who ranged in age from 17 to 67, completed a behavioral treatment either with or without the addition of hypnosis.

At the end of the 9-week program, both interventions resulted in significant weight reduction.

However, *at the 8-month and 2-year follow-ups, the hypnosis clients showed significant additional weight loss*, while those in the behavioral treatment exhibited little further change. More of the subjects who used hypnosis also achieved and maintained their personal weight goals. The utility of employing hypnosis as an adjunct to a behavioral weight-management program is discussed.

---

[3]J Clin Psychol. 1985 Jan;41(1):35-41.

Study: Weight loss for women: studies of smokers and nonsmokers using hypnosis and multicomponent treatments with and without overt aversion.[4]

Another study showing that using Hypnosis for weight loss is effective.

Study 1 compared overweight adult women smokers and nonsmokers in an hypnosis-based, weight-loss program.

Smokers and nonsmokers achieved significant weight losses and decreases in Body Mass Index.

Study 2 treated 100 women either in an hypnosis only or an overt aversion and hypnosis program.

This multicomponent follow-up study replicated significant weight losses and declines in Body Mass Index. The overt aversion and hypnosis program yielded significantly lower posttreatment weights and a greater average number of pounds lost.

Study: Participation in multicomponent hypnosis treatment programs for women's weight loss with and without overt aversion.[5]

Hypnosis was shown to be effective for weight loss.

---

[4]Psychol Rep. 1997 Jun;80(3 Pt 1):931-3.
[5]Psychol Rep. 1996 Oct;79(2):659-68.

Studies of hypnotic, covert and overt aversive techniques have yielded two or more interpretations of results when each has been examined for a singular effect on weight lost. Some have advocated study of effective combinations of techniques before investing in other applications.

Two programs of hypnosis, imagery, diet, tape, behavior management and support but differing in the overt use of aversion (electric shock, disgusting tastes smells) were examined.

A total of 172 overweight adult women were treated, 86 in a hypnosis only and 86 in an overt aversion and hypnosis program. Both programs achieved significant weight losses.

Hypnosis is something that is cheap and easy to incorporate into a weight loss and maintenance plan. There really isn't a reason not to Utilize Hypnosis to help you achieve your weight loss goals and then stay lean for the rest of your life.

Website to order Hypnosis tapes: www.Hypfit.net.

32   Terry

I am not going to identify this person so I will call her Terry. She is the typical female. So I will share some of our conversations so you may learn and maybe even relate. Listening to what Terry says is a perfect example of why I recommend Hypnosis CDs to do along with the protocols in this book. It is also another reason why I recommend reading the book multiple times.

The Hypnosis CDs are something that can be listened to in private on a daily basis. You will see after reading the emails from Terry why Hypnosis is such a good choice to assist with her mindset.

Here is what Terry emailed me after a very short conversation about the book I was writing

Very interested in your book. Told Mike about it. We're proud of you John. I'm sure with all your research it will be a good one. The diet industry is full of harmful and wrong information. The public is so confused and obesity and health is getting worse.

I have not a clue on fasting or how to do it. But I can tell you all about the, Rice Diet, Grapefruit Diet, Low Carb Diet, Weight Watchers, 5 meals a day plan, South Beach diet, Zone, Atkins and let's not forget those diet pills!! I think there is even an ice cream diet. I didn't do that one, it didn't make any sense, a crazy idea!! Although the ones I listed did. I know what your thinking!! Stop that!! Only think kind things about me.

I do have a suggestion for a chapter in your book: Your Self Image. In my case and many other overweight women.

(not sure if this is true with men) My whole life I have thought I was fat. Our family always talked about weight. We were on many different diets as a family. Mom preferred the fruit cocktail and cottage cheese and cantaloupe. If you ate carrots and celery you wouldn't be fat. Most foods make you fat.

As a family we did the Rice Diet and Grapefruit and Calorie counting. I rarely eat with mom today without her talking about each bite of food that goes in her mouth. Dinnertime is a punishment not to be enjoyed.

My sister always told me I was fat in one way or another. When I look at family pictures I was not fat. Now I look like I have always felt. Mom raised two daughters that became obese. Mike understands what I went through. He can't believe how obsessed she is and then he sees her sneaking food all the time. It's really funny during the holidays. She refuses cookies and candies, and then tells us why. Mike and the boys catch her sneaking these foods by the handfuls. On the other hand when I'm really trying to diet she encourages me to eat that piece of pie. "You just have to try it!!"

Not only has the diet industry messed us up, but also we are probably in our 3rd generation of a growing epidemic of obesity and false information.

Americans cannot enjoy eating. Tom said when he traveled in Europe that eating is an event, 7 course meals, wine and conversation. A meal lasts 2 hours. You Americans are too obsessed with diets. They know an American when they see them eating in the car or eating as their walking. You Americans also drink to get drunk. Wine to them was like a glass of milk or water with dinner.

He also was asked "do all American's sue each other to

make money?" At that time his dad was going through that lawsuit and you going through yours. (The IRS terrorized my family and I for 9 years). Then don't get me on the fast food industry. I remember when Bob Dole said cigarettes do not cause cancer. So many lies and misconceptions for the almighty $. Fat people cause insurance to go up. Don't get me on that one. I feel the diet industry and fast food industry had a lot to do with that.

Anyway John, fat people have issues: Why can't I stay on a diet? Many have been raised with a fat or ugly self-image. I was told it takes 10 positives to get rid of one negative. It's so hard to see ourselves and to know ourselves. We don't face the reality of what obesity is doing to our bodies or life. We crave, we eat under stress, eat when we're happy and sad.

We resent being classified as fat and lazy. There are as many lazy skinny people. I created a successful business, laundry done each week, clean house (sometimes cluttered), groceries, etc. I remember Mike and I had 4 jobs between us.

I'm not saying food is not making me fat. I'm saying there are many layers to people. For me I have many layers that have made me who I am. I would really like to take off the many layers that make me fat.

Food is only one of those layers. I'm proud to say I have gotten rid of some of the layers and still working on the others. Your hypnosis could really help for people to peel off those layers. You already know that. My hardest part with hypnosis was not, settling down, not, laughing (nerves) but hearing you say kind things to me. Or trying to get me to think good things about myself. No, I'm not working to get compliments!! Might be a common fact with over weight people. Again that self image.

If you need anymore fat opinions or need to know what it's like being fat just call me.

Writing all about me was not my intention. Just thought my years of experience with feeling fat, raised as fat and being fat might help to give you another idea for a chapter or how about Volume 2 of a future Best Seller!

Love you all!!

Terry

After I read this email, I called her and explained what to do for weight loss. We were on the phone for 3 hours. This took so long because she had so much garbage in her head about dieting. I am including all of this because, there is a very large number of people that are just like Terry, extremely confused about what to do for weight loss.

2nd email

John,

BREAKFAST– Skipping breakfast was not a problem like I thought it would be.

Terry

3rd email

John,

Your information keeps rolling around in my head!!

I have been doing better. Although once the holidays are over, the sugar stuff is out. I know I can have it, it's just that it's a huge red light food for me. I would say during the holidays I've cut way back on snacking and I'm skipping breakfast.

Skipping breakfast seems to give me more energy. I do miss breakfast, but would miss lunch or dinner more.

Wow, you have a lot of interesting chapters. Looks like your covering everything and more. Good job! The first chapter I want to read is "What you learned from Julie". It's gotta be a good one! Mike has requested some pictures in your chapter "Models and Strippers". Go figure.

Have a wonderful Christmas John.

4th email

John my update: After 4 weeks of following your advice I have lost 10 pounds. Not bad! My best weeks are when I skip meals. One day I surprised myself by skipping 2 meals!!! I wasn't hungry all day. A first time in my life experience.

Anyway, it's working for me. I drink more water. I hear dehydration is very common and can make you feel hungry when you really need fluids.

Love you

Terry

I am sure that many of you reading this book can relate to Terry. That is why I included this chapter. There is no reason to be confused about weight loss after reading this book. Terry's mom was confused and she projected her struggles with weight gain onto her children. How much better would all their lives have been if they knew the information in this book?

Remember this, a candle loses nothing by lighting another candle. Share this book with others and free them from the stress of worrying about food. Pay it forward.

33   Fasting History

This is not an all-inclusive list; rather a few examples of some interesting people to show you that fasting has been around a long time.

Hippocrates, the Greek physician who lived around 400 BC, is referred to as the father of Western medicine. Doctors even take a Hippocratic Oath when they graduate which encourages doctors to practice ethically.

Hippocrates was the first person to say that disease is caused from diet, living habits and environmental factors and not caused from superstition or the from the Gods punishment. For his medical views that were against the infrastructure in Greece, he was thrown in prison for 20 years. While in prison he wrote his well-known medical publication called "The Complicated Body" that covered many things we know to be true today. (Yes, sometimes it is no fun to be right, and vocalize your beliefs. I think of the tax protestors of today who courageously argue against government theft of the poor and middle class).

So what kind of advice did Hippocrates give for Obesity?

"Obese people and those desiring to lose weight should perform hard work before food. Meals should be taken after exertion and while still panting from fatigue. *They should, moreover, only eat once per day.*"

So Hippocrates recommended exercising in the fasted state and eating only once per day. As you can see, this advice has been around and working for a long period of time. As I write this book, more and more fitness trainers, dieticians, nutritionists and doctors are once again using the time-tested methods of fasting.

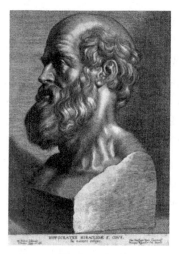

Hippocrates

Dr. Herbert Shelton wrote a book called "The Science and Art of Fasting", which exerted an influence on *Mahatma Gandhi*, who was known to consult the book before undertaking public fasts.

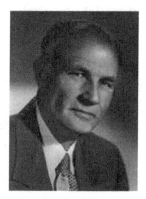

Dr. Herbert Shelton

Dr. Shelton, who attended a Chiropractic College and graduated from a Naturopathic College, had a book published in 1934 called "Fasting and Sunbathing".

This is quite interesting because some of Dr. Shelton's recommendations have really come full circle.

"Fat Loss the Truth", advocates short term fasting (16 to 24 hours primarily) for weight loss and overall health compared to Dr. Shelton's recommendation of much longer periods of fasting (sometimes 30 days).

The second part of his book is about sunbathing. Fast forward to 2011 and nearly every doctor of any worth is testing Vitamin D levels on their patients and recommending more time in the sun, such as sunbathing, and or Vitamin D supplements. It is now known that Vitamin D levels are highly deficient in most of the world and these low levels greatly contribute to increased cancer rates. The research is coming out at a rapid pace on Vitamin D. I encourage you to do a web search for Vitamin D and you will be amazed at the sheer volume of studies that have been completed. Books can be written on this topic alone.

You have to remember that the world was a much different place in the late 1800's and early 1900's than it is now and the level of knowledge and the ability to share knowledge was much different. Just look at the ease of looking up information now on the internet. Dr. Shelton did not have the internet at his fingertips, yet made some very futuristic recommendations that nearly 90 years later, modern research has come to support and some other recommendations that get no support at all.

Shelton was thrown in jail in 1917 for making an anti-draft statement in public. (You have got to like that Dr. Shelton stood for something and there is not much more that a person can support than a peaceful foreign policy initiative and an anti-indentured slavery (forced taxation) stance).

Dr. Shelton was once charged but never tried for starving a patient to death. There have been periods of time in history where people have fasted for long periods of time to improve their health. *Nevertheless, this really has nothing to do with "Fat Loss the Truth", because Shelton's recommendations to not eat for 30 days goes completely against the modern strategies in this book.*

We have not seen a reason in the literature for fasting long periods of time such as 20 to 40 days. After 24 hours of fasting, fat burning starts to slow down.

However, during the 1950's and 1960's there were fasting studies for obesity that involved not eating for long periods of time ranging from 10 days and beyond. One study suggested that a lean person could go approximately 60 – 70 days without eating before dying and an obese person could go 200 – 300 days. In a 1966 study published in the Lancet, 2 obese females fasted for up to 249 days and lost 30% of their bodyweight. The published record for fasting was a man that went 382 days without eating, which was published by Stuart and Flemming in 1973. The 27-year-old man started at 456 lbs and ended up at 180 lbs. He was monitored medically and was given such things as potassium during the fast. He had no ill effects from the fast according to the published study.

To restate what is in this book, "Fat Loss the Truth" recommends repeated short periods of fasting from 16 to 24 hours and does not recommend to fast for days on end. Short periods of fasting are very beneficial to your overall health and are very easy to follow for weight loss.

Another popular person to promote fasting was *Paul Bragg,*

ND.

One of the things Paul Bragg recommended was one 24-hour fast each week.

He also did a 7 to 10 day fast every three months for body purification as he called it.

Bragg advocated taking amino acids. It is funny because here is an example where things come around again and gain popularity again. I quite frequently recommend amino acids to athletes who are fasting and I have seen that some others who are utilizing fasting for fat loss are also recommending amino acids. Let's give credit where credit is due, Bragg was recommending amino acids and fasting in the 1930's, in his book "The Miracle of Fasting."

Here are some of the chapter titles in "The Miracle of Fasting" that you may find interesting: (Just the titles alone have points that remarkably resemble points in the anti-aging movement today):

- No Breakfast Plan is Best (*my note: one of the most popular ways to fast*)

- Juice Fast – an Introduction to Water Fast

- Shorter Fasts Are Better and Safer (*my note: this book only uses short fasts*)

- Fasting Melts Away Pounds!

- Your Waistline is Your Lifeline & Dateline! (my note; the waist measurement has become one of the indicators of Syndrome X in modern medicine)

- Fasting is a Weight Normalizer

- You are as Old as Your Arteries (my note; this statement is now common at anti-aging seminars among cardiologists. I hear it all the time)

- Sunshine Brings Peace, Relaxation to Nerves (my note: obvious Vitamin D recommendations)

- Iodine from Kelp is Important (my note: iodine deficiency has become a hot topic because of it's widespread deficiencies and iodine's requirement for the thyroid gland which helps regulate metabolism)

- Should You Exercise While Fasting? (*my note: exercise while fasting burns more body fat than exercise after eating*)

- Iron Pumping (my note: research is now supporting weight lifting for maintaining your metabolism and muscle. Doctors now even recommend weightlifting to prevent osteoporosis)

- Amazing Strength Results in 8 Weeks (my note: this is now common in studies and advertising showing before and after results)

Those chapter headlines really ring true today. Do we know more today than Bragg did in 1930. Of course we do. It's kind of like automobiles. Compare an auto of today with one from 1930. There have been advancements obviously.

Many celebrities have followed Bragg's health recommendations including actors and musicians. It is undeniable that he inspired many people.

However, Bragg was not without controversy. It has been argued that Bragg was not nearly as old as he claimed. Many believe that he was actually 14 years younger than he claimed and that he claimed he was much older as a way of promoting his business.

When you first look at some of these older books by Shelton and Bragg from nearly a century ago, some of their recommendations seem flat out ridiculous (they most likely are), but I kept an open mind and decided to see what else I could find to support some of their stuff.

As it turns out, they both said many things that are proving true today. Kind of like if you compared the first airplane at Kittyhawk to a modern stealth fighter, if we didn't have that first plane that barely got off the ground, we wouldn't have the crazy fast jets we have today.

Jack LaLanne was an American fitness icon

Jack LaLanne got his start being interested in health after his mother took him to a health and nutrition seminar put on by Paul Bragg, ND.

Jack was a Doctor of Chiropractic who had a television show "The Jack LaLanne Show" that ran for 34 years. He has invented fitness equipment, started a chain of health clubs and sold juicers on infomercials.

Jack has performed many fitness feats such as; while handcuffed and shackled, he swam 1.5 miles towing 70 boats with 70 people at age 70. Nearly his whole life he has exercised 2 hours per day as part of his lifestyle.

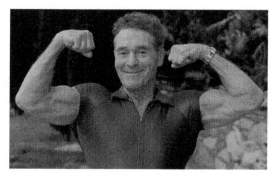

Jack LaLanne age 71

Jack would take large doses of vitamins, minerals, herbs and enzymes. He got protein from eggs and fish. He ate brown rice and whole wheat, 5-6 pieces of fresh fruit and 10 raw vegetables a day. He never ate dessert and *never ate past 9 pm.*

So what did Jack LaLanne say about weight loss?

Here are a few pieces of an interview on the Larry King show from July 17th, 2000: (edited for length)

KING: Dunseth, North Dakota – Hello.

CALLER: *Hello, how does a 300-pound woman start an exercise program?*

LA LANNE: Get a physical. That's very important for a lot of people who haven't exercised for long to get a physical and find out what your blood pressure and everything is. *The No. 1 thing, if you are overweight, you have to count calories – period.* (This is another example of the main point of Fat Loss the Truth; *calorie restriction is the main point for weight loss*)

KING: In other words, if you just exercise, it ain't going to work.

LA LANNE: Oh, absolutely not. You can't do that much exercise.

Jack gives more pointers from an interview with Donald Katz in 1995

I asked Jack LaLanne if he ever snacks before bedtime.

"Never!" he snarled. "You don't get it. I am one runaway son of a bitch! I am an animal! I want to eat everything! I want to get drunk every single night! I want to screw every woman there is! We are all wild animals. But we must learn to use our minds. We must learn to control the bestial and sensual sides of ourselves!"

Here's some more advice on exercise and diet given by Jack LaLanne in an interview with Share Guide.

Share Guide: What would you tell a beginner? (about exercise)

Jack LaLanne: The main thing is to start a weight-training program. Also, you should change your program every 30 days. That's the key.

Another tidbit from Jack: One thing you have to remember is Scales Lie! The biggest liars we have are the scales. I always ask in my lectures, "What did you weigh when you were 20 years old?" Someone will say, "Oh, I weighed 170 lbs." But then they played football and basketball, and were in good shape. Now the guy is 50 years old and he says, "Jack, I haven't gained a pound! I weigh 170 just like I did when I was 20!" I'll say "Really, that's wonderful! How big was your waist when you were 20?" "Oh, 30 inches" "How big is it today?" "Oh, 36." The sands of time have shifted. The guy put five or six inches on his waist. You figure about every inch is five pounds approximately. That guy has gained about 30 pounds of fat and lost 30 pounds of muscle and the scale says he weighs the same.

Share Guide: So it's what you are made of not how much you weigh.

Jack LaLanne: Yes. What you need to do is get that tape measure out, and start measuring that gut. Then, you start working out and you start eating properly till that gut gets down close to where it was when you were in your 20's. Then you'll find out what your weight should be.

Share Guide: *Haven't you said you never snack?*

Jack LaLanne: *Never. Only water between meals.*

Share Guide: What do you think about the current low-carb craze?

Jack LaLanne: It's a bunch of bull!...One guy says don't mix carbohydrates, and the other guy says don't mix protein with it; it's a bunch of lard, something to sell a book. And *the poor public is so confused; they don't know what to do.*

Here are studies that show Calorie Restriction and Fasting can be used for more things than just weight loss. Apparently, some more of the things that were said about fasting so long ago are turning out to be true: To make this easy to understand, my notes are at the beginning and are shaded.

Study: Fasting and differential chemotherapy protection in patients.[1]

Fasting reduced side effects from chemotherapy.

Chronic calorie restriction has been known for decades to prevent or retard cancer growth, but its weight-loss effect and the potential problems associated with combining it with chemotherapy have prevented its clinical application.

Based on the discovery in model organisms that fasting causes a rapid switch of cells to a protected mode, we described a fasting-based intervention that causes remarkable changes in the levels of glucose, IGF-I and many other proteins and molecules and is capable of protecting mammalian cells and mice from various toxins, including chemotherapy.

Because oncogenes prevent the cellular switch to this stress resistance mode, starvation for 48 hours or longer protects normal yeast and mammalian cells and mice but not cancer cells from chemotherapy, an effect we termed Differential Stress Resistance (DSR).

In a recent article, *10 patients who fasted in combination with chemotherapy, reported that fasting was not only feasible and safe but caused a reduction in a wide range of side effects accompanied by an apparently normal and possibly augmented chemotherapy efficacy.*

Together with the remarkable results observed in animals, these data provide preliminary evidence in support

---

[1]Giannina Gaslini Institute; Genova, Italy. Cell Cycle. 2010 Nov 15;9(22):4474-4476.

of the human application of this fundamental biogeron-
tology finding, particularly for terminal patients receiving chemotherapy. Here we briefly discuss the basic, pre-
clinical, and clinical studies on fasting and cancer therapy.

Study: Impact of 6-month caloric restriction on autonomic nervous system activity in healthy, overweight, individuals.[2]

Calorie Restriction and exercise utilized together improved the nervous system.

Caloric restriction (CR) increases maximum lifespan but
the mechanisms are unclear. Dominance of the sympathetic nervous system (SNS) over the parasympathetic nervous system (PNS) has been shown to be a strong risk factor for cardiovascular disease.

Obesity and aging are associated with increased SNS activity, and weight loss and/or exercise seem to have positive
effects on this balance.

We therefore evaluated the effect of different approaches
of Calorie Restriction on autonomic function in 28 overweight individuals participating in the Comprehensive Assessment of Long-term Effects of Reducing Intake of Energy (CALERIE) trial.

Participants were randomized to either:

- control,

[2]Pennington Biomedical Research Center, Louisiana State University System, Baton Rouge, Louisiana, USA. Obesity (Silver Spring).
2010 Feb;18(2):414-6. Epub 2009 Nov 12.

- CR: 25% decrease in energy intake,

- CREX: 12.5% CR + 12.5% increase in energy expenditure,

- LCD: low-calorie diet until 15% weight reduction followed by weight maintenance.

Autonomic function was assessed by spectral analysis of heart-rate variability (HRV) while fasting and after a meal.

The results suggest that weight loss improved SNS/PNS balance especially when Calorie Restriction is combined with exercise.

Study: Calorie restriction and bone health in young, overweight individuals.[3]

People that did calorie restriction for 6 months lost over 10% of their bodyweight and their bones remained strong.

Methods: Forty-six individuals were randomized to 4 groups for 6 months:

1. healthy diet (control group)

2. 25% Calorie Restriction from baseline energy requirements (CR group)

[3]Pennington Comprehensive Assessment of Long-Term Effects of Reducing Intake of Energy (CALERIE) Research Team. Collaborators (18); Pennington Biomedical Research Center, Baton Rouge, LA 70808, USA. Arch Intern Med. 2008 Sep 22;168(17):1859-66.

3. 25% energy deficit by a combination of Calorie Restriction and increased aerobic exercise (CR + EX group)

4. low-calorie diet (890 kcal/d; goal, 15% weight loss) followed by weight maintenance (LCD group).

Bone mineral density and serum bone markers were measured at baseline and after 6 months.

Results:

Mean body weight was reduced by:

- 1.0% (control)

- 10.4% (CR)

- 10.0% (CR + EX)

- 13.9% (LCD)

Compared with the control group, none of the groups showed any change in bone mineral density for total body or hip.

Study: Dietary factors, hormesis and health.[4]

Fasting reduces calorie intake which protects against disease and increases lifespan.

The impact of dietary factors on health and longevity is increasingly appreciated. The most prominent dietary factor

[4]Laboratory of Neurosciences, National Institute on Aging Intramural Research Program, Baltimore, MD 21224, USA. Ageing Res Rev. 2008 Jan;7(1):43-8. Epub 2007 Sep 1.

that affects the risk of many different chronic diseases is energy intake – excessive calorie intake increases the risk.

Reducing energy intake by controlled caloric restriction or intermittent fasting increases lifespan and protects various tissues against disease, in part, by hormesis mechanisms that increase cellular stress resistance.

Study: Caloric restriction and aging as viewed from Biosphere2[5]

Calorie Restriction improved the overall health of these people.

The low-calorie nutrient-dense diet consumed for 2 years by the eight persons sealed inside the closed ecological space known as Biosphere 2, near Tucson, AZ, constituted a unique "experiment of nature," amounting to the first well-monitored application of a nutritional regimen proven in animals to substantially inhibit and delay time of onset of most age-related diseases, induce physiological changes characteristic of a functionally "younger" age, and extend both average and maximum lifespans.

Over the 2 years the eight persons demonstrated a substantial weight loss, remarkable fall in blood cholesterol, blood pressure, fasting blood sugar, and low white blood cell counts–exactly as seen in rodents on such a regimen.

---

[5]Department of Pathology, UCLA School of Medicine, USA. Receptor. 1995 Spring;5(1):29-33.

Study: Short-term modified alternate-day fasting: a novel dietary strategy for weight loss and cardioprotection in obese adults.[6]

Alternate day fasting caused a constant rate of weight loss, improved indicators for coronary artery disease and to top it off with good news; obese people followed the fasting plan.

Background: The ability of modified alternate-day fasting (ADF; ie, consuming 25% of energy needs on the fast day and ad libitum (at one's pleasure) food intake on the following day) to facilitate weight loss and lower vascular disease risk in obese individuals remains unknown.

Objective: This study examined the effects of ADF that is administered under controlled compared with self-implemented conditions on body weight and coronary artery disease (CAD) risk indicators in obese adults.

Design: Sixteen obese subjects (12 women, 4 men) completed a 10-week trial, which consisted of 3 phases:

1. a 2-week control phase

2. a 4-week weight loss/ADF controlled food intake phase

3. a 4-week weight loss/ADF self-selected food intake phase.

---

[6]Department of Kinesiology and Nutrition, University of Illinois at Chicago, Chicago, IL 60612, USA. Am J Clin Nutr. 2009 Nov;90(5):1138-43. Epub 2009 Sep 30.

Results: *Dietary adherence remained high* throughout the controlled food intake phase (days adherent: 86%) and the self-selected food intake phase (days adherent: 89%).

The rate of weight loss remained constant during controlled food intake (0.67 +/- 0.1 kg/wk) and self-selected food intake phases (0.68 +/- 0.1 kg/wk).

Total cholesterol, LDL cholesterol, and triacylglycerol concentrations decreased, respectively, after 8 week of ADF. Systolic blood pressure decreased.

Conclusion: These findings suggest that ADF is a viable diet option to help obese individuals lose weight and decrease CAD risk.

Study: Caloric restriction: from soup to nuts.[7]

Calorie Restriction studies show improved longevity in many different species.

Caloric restriction (CR), reduced protein, methionine, or tryptophan diets; and reduced insulin and/or IGFI intracellular signaling *can extend mean and/or maximum lifespan and delay deleterious age-related physiological changes* in animals.

Many health benefits are induced by even brief periods of CR in flies, rodents, monkeys, and humans. In humans and nonhuman primates, CR produces most of the physiologic, hematologic, hormonal, and biochemical changes it produces in other animals.

[7]Department of Biochemistry, University of California, Riverside, Riverside, CA, USA. Ageing Res Rev. 2010 Jul;9(3):324-53. Epub 2009 Oct 21.

In primates, *Calorie Restriction provides protection from type 2 diabetes, cardiovascular and cerebral vascular diseases, immunological decline, malignancy, hepatotoxicity, liver fibrosis and failure, sarcopenia, inflammation, and DNA damage.* It also enhances muscle mitochondrial biogenesis, affords neuroprotection; and extends mean and maximum lifespan.

Study: Calorie restriction extends Saccharomyces cerevisiae lifespan by increasing respiration.[8]

Calorie restriction is the only regimen known to lengthen the lifespan of mammals and respiration (metabolism) actually increases.

Calorie restriction (CR) extends lifespan in a wide spectrum of organisms and *is the only regimen known to lengthen the lifespan of mammals.* We established a model of CR in budding yeast Saccharomyces cerevisiae. In this study we explore how CR activates Sir2 to extend lifespan. Here we show that the shunting of carbon metabolism toward the mitochondrial tricarboxylic acid cycle and the concomitant increase in respiration play a central part in this process.

---

[8]Department of Biology, Massachusetts Institute of Technology, Cambridge, Massachusetts 02139, USA. Nature. 2002 Jul 18;418(6895):344-8.

Study: Calorie restriction induces mitochondrial biogenesis and bioenergetic efficiency.[9]

The mitochondria are the energy plants in your cells. When using calorie restriction, there is less wear and tear on your energy plants and at the same time they still keep making energy called ATP.

Age-related accumulation of cellular damage and death has been linked to oxidative stress. *Calorie restriction (CR) is the most robust, nongenetic intervention that increases lifespan and reduces the rate of aging in a variety of species.* Mechanisms responsible for the anti aging effects of CR remain uncertain, but reduction of oxidative stress within mitochondria remains a major focus of research. Moreover, mitochondria *under CR conditions* show less oxygen consumption, reduce membrane potential, and *generate less reactive oxygen species (bad stuff that damages your body) than controls, but remarkably they are able to maintain their critical ATP production.*

---

[9]Centro Andaluz de Biología del Desarrollo, Universidad Pablo de Olavide, 41013 Sevilla, Spain. Proc Natl Acad Sci U S A. 2006 Feb 7;103(6):1768-73. Epub 2006 Jan 30.

Study: Caloric restriction promotes genomic stability by induction of base excision repair and reversal of its age-related decline.[10]

Calorie Restriction helps repair DNA.

Caloric restriction is a potent experimental manipulation that extends mean and maximum life span and *delays the onset and progression of tumors* in laboratory rodents.

We provide evidence that CR promotes genomic stability *by increasing DNA repair capacity, specifically base excision repair (BER). CR completely reverses the age-related decline in BER capacity in all tissues tested (brain, liver, spleen and testes).*

Study: Beneficial effects of intermittent fasting and caloric restriction on the cardiovascular and cerebrovascular systems.[11]

Fasting improves cardiovascular and brain functions among other things.

Intermittent fasting (IF; reduced meal frequency) and caloric restriction (CR) extend lifespan and increase resis-

---

[10]Department of Nutrition and Food Science, Wayne State University, 3009 Science Hall, Detroit, MI 48202, USA. DNA Repair (Amst). 2003 Mar 1;2(3):295-307.

[11]Laboratory of Neurosciences, National Institute on Aging Intramural Research Program, Baltimore, MD 21224, USA. J Nutr Biochem. 2005 Mar;16(3):129-37.

tance to age-related diseases in rodents and monkeys and improve the health of overweight humans.

Both IF and CR *enhance cardiovascular and brain functions and improve several risk factors for coronary artery disease and stroke including a reduction in blood pressure and increased insulin sensitivity.*

The beneficial effects of IF and CR result from at least two mechanisms–reduced oxidative damage and increased cellular stress resistance.

Interestingly, cellular and molecular effects of IF and CR on the cardiovascular system and the brain are similar to those of regular physical exercise, suggesting shared mechanisms.

Study: Cardioprotection by intermittent fasting in rats.[12]

Fasting helps your heart.

Background: We have reported neuroprotective effects of IF (intermittent fasting) against ischemic injury of the brain. In this study, we examined the effects of IF on ischemic injury of the heart in rats.

Conclusions: *Intermittent Fasting protects the heart from ischemic injury and attenuates post-myocardial infaction cardiac remodeling,* likely via antiapoptotic and antiinflammatory mechanisms.

---

[12]Laboratory of Cardiovascular Sciences, National Institute on Aging, Intramural Research Program, National Institutes of Health, Baltimore, MD, USA. Circulation. 2005 Nov 15;112(20):3115-21. Epub 2005 Nov 7.

Study: Caloric restriction and intermittent fasting alter spectral measures of heart rate and blood pressure variability in rats.[13]

Fasting improved blood pressure, heart rate and body weight.

Dietary restriction (DR) has been shown to increase life span, delay or prevent age-associated diseases, and improve functional and metabolic cardiovascular risk factors in rodents and other species. To investigate the effects of DR on beat-to-beat heart rate and diastolic blood pressure variability (HRV and DPV) in rats, we implanted telemetric transmitters and animals were maintained on either intermittent fasting (every other day feeding) or calorie-restricted (40% caloric reduction) diets.

Using power spectral analysis, we evaluated the temporal profiles of the low- and high-frequency oscillatory components in heart rate and diastolic blood pressure signals to assess cardiac autonomic activity. *Body weight, heart rate, and systolic and diastolic blood pressure were all found to decrease in response to Dietary Restriction.* Both methods of DR produced decreases in the low-frequency component of DPV spectra, a marker for sympathetic tone, and the high-frequency component of HRV spectra, a marker for parasympathetic activity, was increased. These parameters required at least 1 month to become maximal, but returned toward baseline values rapidly once rats resumed

[13]Laboratory of Neurosciences, National Institute on Aging, 5600 Nathan Shock Dr, Baltimore, MD 21224, USA. FASEB J. 2006 Apr;20(6):631-7.

ad libitum diets. These results suggest an additional cardiovascular benefit of DR that merits further studies of this potential effect in humans.

Study: Dietary protein restriction decreases oxidative protein damage, peroxidizability index, and mitochondrial complex I content in rat liver.[14]

Calorie Restriction slows the aging rate but neither carb nor fat restriction alone has been shown to extend life. Studies such as this may provide information about improved ways to fast in the future.

Caloric restriction (CR) decreases oxidative damage, which contributes to the slowing of aging rate. It is not known if such decreases are due to calories themselves or specific dietary components. In this work, the ingestion of proteins of rats was decreased by 40% below that of controls.

After 7 weeks, *the liver of the protein-restricted (PR) animals showed decreases in oxidative protein damage, degree of membrane unsaturation, and mitochondrial complex I content.*

Recent studies suggest that those benefits of PR could be caused, in turn, by the lowered methionine intake of that dietary manipulation.

---

[14]Department of Basic Medical Sciences, Faculty of Medicine, University of Lleida, Spain. J Gerontol A Biol Sci Med Sci. 2007 Apr;62(4):352-60.

Study: Mitochondrial oxidative stress, aging and caloric restriction: the protein and methionine connection.[15]

Reducing specific amino acids like methionine may become an important point after more research is completed in the future. Time will tell.

Caloric restriction (CR) decreases aging rate and mitochondrial ROS (MitROS) production and oxidative stress in rat postmitotic tissues. Low levels of these parameters are also typical traits of long-lived mammals and birds. However, it is not known what dietary components are responsible for these changes during CR. It was recently observed that 40% protein restriction without strong CR also decreases MitROS generation and oxidative stress. This is interesting because *protein restriction also increases maximum longevity (although to a lower extent than Calorie Restriction)* and is a much more practicable intervention for humans than CR.

Moreover, it was recently found that 80% methionine restriction substituting it for l-glutamate in the diet also decreases MitROS generation in rat liver. Thus, methionine restriction seems to be responsible for the decrease in ROS production observed in caloric restriction.

This is interesting because it is known that exactly that procedure of methionine restriction also increases maximum longevity. Moreover, recent data show that methionine levels in tissue proteins negatively correlate with maximum

---

[15]Department of Basic Medical Sciences, University of Lleida, Lleida 25008, Spain. Biochim Biophys Acta. 2006 May-Jun;1757(5-6):496-508. Epub 2006 Feb 24.

longevity in mammals and birds. All these suggest that lowering of methionine levels is involved in the control of mitochondrial oxidative stress and vertebrate longevity by at least two different mechanisms: decreasing the sensitivity of proteins to oxidative damage, and lowering of the rate of ROS generation at mitochondria.

Study: Short-term fasting in normal women: absence of effects on gonadotrophin secretion and the menstrual cycle.[16]

Female Hormones remained normal while Fasting.

In this study we investigated the effects of a short-term fast (72 hours) on female reproductive hormone secretion and menstrual function.

Patients: Eight normal cycling women, ages 21-35, within 10% of ideal body weight, were fasted for 72 hours during the follicular phase of their menstrual cycle.

Measurements: On the admission day, the last day of the fast and the day of refeeding, blood samples were collected at 10-minute intervals from 0800 to 2000 hours for determination of the LH pulse pattern. Daily determinations of immuno LH, FSH, oestradiol (E) and progesterone (P) were performed throughout the menstrual cycle in which the fast occurred.

Results: The short-term fast did not have discernible effects upon the reproductive hormones studied. Basal mean

---

[16]Department of Obstetrics and Gynecology, University of Washington, Seattle. Clin Endocrinol (Oxf). 1994 Jun;40(6):725-31. Clin Endocrinol (Oxf). 1994 Jun;40(6):725-31.

LH concentrations did not show any significant variation throughout the study period. Each woman maintained a physiological pattern of LH, FSH, E and P throughout the menstrual cycle including the LH surge; ultrasound evidence of normal growth of a dominant follicle; and cycle length consistent with previous cycles.

Conclusions: *Our results indicate that in spite of profound metabolic changes, a 72-hour fast during the follicular phase does not affect the menstrual cycle of normal cycling women.*

Study: Short-term fasting induces profound neuronal autophagy.[17]

Fasting repairs the nervous system.

Disruption of autophagy–a key homeostatic process in which cytosolic components are degraded and recycled through lysosomes–can cause neurodegeneration in tissue culture and in vivo.

Upregulation of this pathway may be neuroprotective, and much effort is being invested in developing drugs that cross the blood brain barrier and increase neuronal autophagy. *One well-recognized way of inducing autophagy is by food restriction,* which upregulates autophagy in many organs including the liver.

We use the method to identify constitutive autophagosomes in cortical neurons and Purkinje cells, and *we show*

---

[17]Department of Immunology and Microbial Science, The Scripps Research Institute, La Jolla, CA, USA. Autophagy. 2010 Aug 16;6(6):702-10. Epub 2010 Aug 14.

that short-term fasting leads to a dramatic upregulation in neuronal autophagy.

Our data lead us to speculate that sporadic *fasting might represent a simple, safe and inexpensive means to promote this potentially therapeutic neuronal response.*

34   Final Thought

Here is the thing; I encourage you to read this book over and over to keep yourself reminded of the scientific facts that have been brought to your attention with this book.

Read through the book again and again, a few pages each day. Keep doing this as many times as it takes until it is a part of you. I fully expect to get emails telling me "I have read your book 20 times." *This will keep you focused and on track.*

You will be bombarded with people, magazines, commercials for food and many other onslaughts of material that can cloud your mind if you let it.

Remember the facts are right in front of you in this book.

You have read thru the book, now get started immediately by skipping meals.

I Have One Request

If this book changes your life, gives you dietary freedom or any other big benefits, buy a copy for someone else and help them succeed also.

What To Look For In The Future

I am currently working on the follow up book to this. It will not replace this book. It is an add on book that covers additional information and topics for those of you who want specifics like, how to check yourself for free for food sensitivities, how to do some self checks for your thyroid gland and tips on how to optimize your diet to look better and feel great.

Final Thought

Thank you for reading this book.

Spread love over hate, Good over evil and Light over darkness. Visualize a white light filling your body and surrounding the planet every day. I promise you will feel better and help everyone by doing this.

Peace, Love and Light

Now, set this book down in a place where you will remember to start reading at the beginning of the book again tomorrow.

Picture Page And Quotes

I work with many athletes and other celebrities. Due to space limitations I only have included a few pictures. I am sorry if I didn't include you if you are reading this, but I had a space limit. I still like you ☺

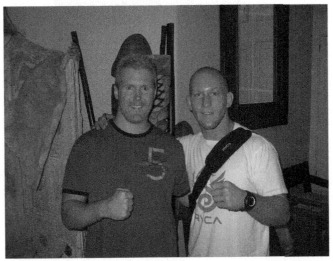

Dr. John Fitzgerald and Gray Maynard, famous MMA Fighter.

"Being a professional athlete, I need to take care of my body. Since I have been working with John, I perform better and recover better. He is really good at what he does and after you have talked with him for 5 minutes you know you are with someone who is not only the best, but he will bend over backward to help you"

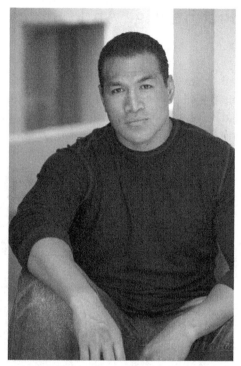

Ray Sefo, 6-time World kick boxing champion from New Zealand, actor and businessman.

"John Fitzgerald really helped me understand the reason why I should take supplements as a professional athlete. Every time I talk to him I learn something. I have seen him the last 3 years and he is one of the reasons I am still fighting at a high level at 40 years old. Thanks for all you help doc!!"

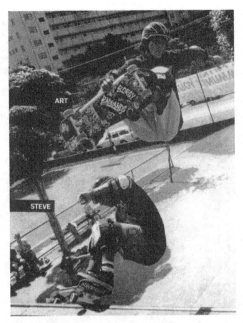

Art and Steve Godoy, famous skateboarders who are still living
on the edge in their 40's. They have also invented tattoo
equipment.

"We want to be doing the same activities we have enjoyed
since we were kids until we die...skateboarding, surfing,
tattooing, playing guitar/drums in a punk band and of
course women...and yea, it is possible with the correct
mindset and full attention to our health needs. Doctor
John knows from experience what the body needs to keep
up our lifestyles all the way down to the cellular level.

Whether you fight for a living or just wanna keep what you
have, it all starts with nutrition. Dr. John helped cure Arts
frozen shoulders, improve our stamina on half pipes and
pools, on waves, on stage and with women all starting with
adopting simple nutritional practices. Hail John Fitzgerald"

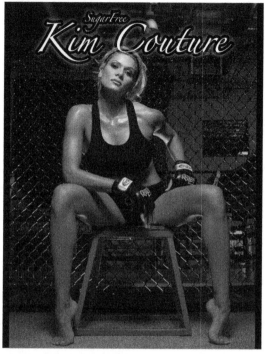

Kim Couture, Pro MMA fighter and business entrepreneur.

"As a Pro Athlete, the information about health and nutrition is obviously a priority to me! After meeting and working with Dr. John Fitzgerald very closely, my body as far as weight loss, recovery and performance changed dramatically! I am now at the age of 35 and 2 children later, in the best shape of my life and still competing Professionally with the Best of them , Thanks to his help and knowledge!"

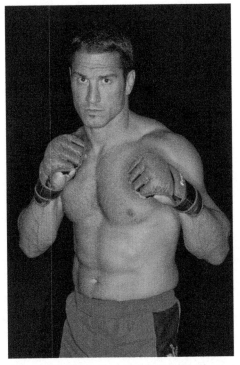

Guy Mezger, UFC Champion, 5-time World Champion, and President of HD Net Fights.

"I really wish that I had met Dr. Fitzgerald early in my athletic career versus the end. He has been crucial in helping stay at my physical best (even in retirement). Dr. Fitzgerald's advice and wisdom is something all of us should take to heart."

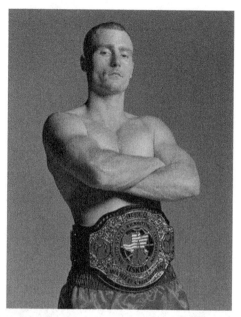

Tim "Bring the Pain" Lane USKBA Super Lightweight World Kickboxing Champion. Tim trains many pro athletes as well as actors and musicians.

"Dr. Fitzgerald has helped restore my body and has given me the energy and vitality I had when I was competing as a fighter. When I was 35, I retired after competing for over 25 years. My energy levels and body were not what they used to be. I transitioned from a professional full time fighter to a professional coach and full time trainer and instructor. It was then that a pro fighter introduced me to Dr. Fitzgerald. He gave me the energy that I had in my teens and 20s. I feel just like I did then – that I can do anything and conquer all! I can't believe how lean I am again without really even setting that as a goal. It just happened."

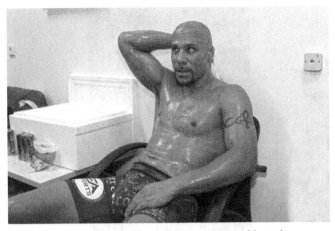

Frank Trigg, famous MMA fighter, actor and broadcaster.

"When I first went to John it was to get stronger and to lose some body fat. What really was the problem was that I had a ton of joint pain that was affecting my training. John listened to what I wanted and learned what I really needed. Now I train everyday stronger and faster with less body fat and no joint pain!! I think John can make anyone rethink their beliefs in one conversation. I thought I knew what to eat as an athlete; I even have a close friend who studied nutrition at an Ivy League college. John told me a better way. I like to check on what he says with my friend. As it turned out, the research supported exactly what John said and not what my Ivy League friend said. I know when I ask John something, I am going to get a straightforward honest answer for sure and that is why so many pros from around the country call on him when they have a question. He is one of those rare people who have a lot of knowledge and at the same time will tell you the truth".

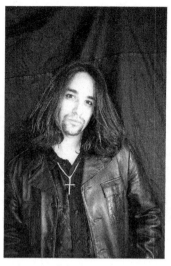

Richard Moreno, owner of the legendary School of Rock in Las Vegas.

"I had been struggling with my weight since I reached my mid 40's. My weight had crept up about 30 lbs. I was focused on eating. I felt I had to eat all the time to lose weight. I spoke with John for about 30 minutes and mostly what he did was ask me questions. The light bulb went off in my head. His advice was so simple yet so effective. Now I don't eat breakfast, sometimes I don't each lunch also when I am busy. I eat after all the bands for the day have practiced. I feel better and it makes my day so much easier. My weight crept right back down and all my clothes fit well again. There are some high level people who bring their kids to the School of Rock and the person that sticks out the most is John. You know there is something special about him. When he talked to me about fat loss, I couldn't stop thinking about it for the next week. It seems like I didn't really do anything and the body fat is gone"

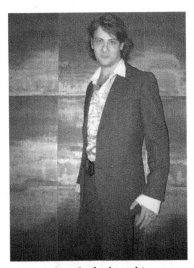

Igor Ledochowski
Co-founder of Street Hypnosis Publishing
www.streethypnosis.com

"I met Dr. John Fitzgerald through a mutual friend, and I am VERY glad that I did. In a world filled with double talk no one understands or people that totally contradict each other about nutrition, it was great to hear someone give simple advice that really worked! John has a way of cutting through all the complexities and half truths and letting you know where you stand. He opened my eyes to just how bad for you most processed or packaged foods can be. At the time I had problems with my adrenal glands and poor digestion, in part due to a hard travel schedule and a growing bad habit of eating "convenience foods." John really helped me out: in a few months, with some simple diet changes and without changing anything in my work schedule, everything was fixed. He even caught and helped me fix an issue which could have led to cancer had it been left unchecked!"

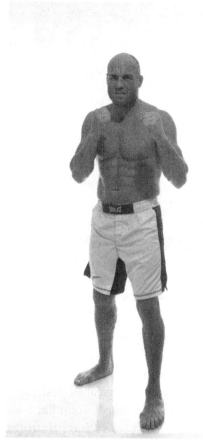

Randy Couture, 6-time UFC Champion and Hall of Famer, actor.

"John Fitzgerald has been working with me personally on getting the most out of my body physically for five years now. My work with him has resulted in a top-notch supplement line and has allowed me longevity into my late 40's in the most demanding sport in professional athletics!"

Thank you to my proofreaders: Julie Fitzgerald, Colton Fitzgerald, Amy Robinson, Mike Anderson, Marco Rafalovich, Ron, Jed and Chito.

Made in the USA
Middletown, DE
28 June 2022